ON THE NOTION OF MENTAL ILLNESS

On the Notion of Mental Illness

Problematizing the medical-model conception of certain abnormal behaviour and mental afflictions

TOMMY SVENSSON

Avebury

Aldershot • Brookfield USA • Hong Kong • Singapore • Sydney

Published by
Avebury
Ashgate Publishing Limited
Gower House
Croft Road
Aldershot
Hants GU11 3HR
England

Ashgate Publishing Company
Old Post Road
Brookfield
Vermont 05036
USA

British Library Cataloguing in Publication Data

Svensson, Tommy
On the Notion of Mental Illness: Problematizing the Medical-Model Conception of Certain Abnormal Behaviour and Mental Afflictions. - (Avebury Series in Philosophy)
I. Title II. Series
616.89001

ISBN 1 85972 160 5

Library of Congress Catalog Card Number: 95-78042

Printed and bound in Great Britain by
Ipswich Book Co. Ltd., Ipswich, Suffolk

Contents

Preface

This book is a revised version of my doctoral thesis, published in 1990 in the series Linköping Studies in Arts and Science. The contents have been restructured, some parts of the text have been substantially rewritten and new text has been added, especially in chapters 5 and 6. I have tried to consider some of the critical comments I received on the earlier version.

A number of persons have, in various ways, been helpful. I have benefited a lot from discussions with three philosophers: Lennart Nordenfelt, Bo Peterson and Ingmar Pörn. Anton Aggernaes, Johan Cullberg, and Göran Eberhard supplied constructive criticism from the point of view of the discipline of psychiatry. With my fellow-sociologist Jan-Håkan Hansson I have had numerous discussions concerning the subject area of the book and he also read and commented on a late version of the manuscript. Malcolm Forbes improved my English and Monika Thörnell assisted in the preparation of the camera ready copy. Needless to say I take the full responsibility for all remaining errors in the book. Special thanks are due to my family, Lena and Jakob, for their encouragement and support.

I gratefully acknowledge financial support from the Bank of Sweden Tercentenary Foundation.

Linköping in May 1995

Tommy Svensson

1 On the whys and hows of discussing the medical-model conception of abnormal behaviour and mental afflictions

Background and introduction

Introductory notes on the plan and structure of this study

This study inquires into some polemics concerning the notion of mental illness or disease.[1] It takes its point of departure in the contention that the case against the medical-model conception of certain abnormal behaviour and mental afflictions was prematurely closed, and that there are good reasons for returning to, for reviving, and for reappraising some central arguments in the debate on psychiatry, and on the psychiatric discourse on human and social problems, of the late 1960's and early 70's. The main purpose of the inquiry is to assess the strength of some parts of the criticism of the concept of mental illness.

The study is divided into six chapters. Chapter 1 is intended to convey a sense of, and provide some arguments in favour of, the need of revitalizing some of the more theoretically inclined arguments against the mental-illness notion. The chapter provides some overviews and characterizations of the early debate, and it includes some methodological deliberations. Chapters 2-5 contain the main analyses and arguments of the study. The analysis of the strengths of the critique, and of some counter-critical strategies, is performed in two steps. In chapters 2 and 3 some fairly well-known elements in the theoretically founded criticism of the notion of mental illness or disease, and some often referred to objections to this criticism, are made the object of discussion in the context of an analysis of the polemics surrounding Thomas Szasz's criticism of psychiatry. In chapters 4 and 5 the analysis is taken further. The Szaszian type of critique is tested against two articulate and up-to-date medical models, with the intent of trying out the possibilities of problematizing the applications of those models to so-called mental-illness phenomena. Chapter 6, finally, includes some comments and reflections on extra-theoretical arguments for and against the medical-model conception of abnormal behaviour and mental afflictions. The chapter also contains some suggestions as to how an ideological analysis of that conception could be undertaken.

The debate on psychiatry: Yesterday and today

Current discussions of psychiatry and psychiatry-related issues differ substantially from the intense debate that flourished 20-25 years ago. The changes that have taken place could be described as shifts along a number of dimensions: from matters of theory to matters of practice, from clashes of contradictory paradigms and perspectives to eclecticism, from openly stated politically motivated conflict to apolitical consensus, from revolutionary demands for immediate and radical changes to precautious and modest ambitions concerning long-term development, etc.

These changes are probably connected to, or expressions of, a major change in the political and ideological climate, that pervades discussion on almost all levels of discourse in Western society. The heated debate on psychiatry of the 1960's and early 70's took place, and could only be comprehended, within the context of a broad and multi-faceted critique of many established ideas, institutional practices and taken-for-granted ways of thinking about and dealing with human and social affairs, but such a critique is lacking today.

The questions that are still asked with regard to psychiatry-related issues are of a quite different nature, and they are asked in a different tone, than was the case during the late 60's and early 70's. And, which is perhaps the most noteworthy, some questions are not asked at all today.

The early debate, in retrospect, seems somewhat confusing and not self-evidently easy to analyze. There are, I believe, several reasons for this. One obviously complicating factor in such an analysis is the variety of aspects of psychiatric theory and practice that the critique was directed against. There was a questioning of specific elements of psychiatric practice. There was, for instance, a turning against certain treatment strategies, such as electroshock treatment, psycho-surgery and the massive use of drugs, that to many critics seemed brutal and primitive ways of dealing with human problems. There was a questioning the fact that psychiatric institutional care and custody in most countries formed a special organizational set-up, separated from the rest of the health-care system, with separate hospitals and a separate legislation concerning the legal status of mental patients. This, to some critics, seemed to express an out-dated segregational attitude. The societal functions of psychiatric practice and theory were questioned, and a prominent feature of much sociologically oriented criticism was the notion that psychiatry in fact primarily performes a social-control function that has very little to do with medical matters. Yet another line of criticism focused on the seemingly ever-continuing expansion of the area of human and social problems that psychiatry claimed to possess the legitimate expertise for handling, theoretically as well as practically. Psychiatric thought-models and therapeutic efforts seemed to be applicable to an almost unlimited range of human predicaments in a way that, it was suggested, threatened to medicalize our lives and our views of reality to an extent where morals and politics would become completely obscured by an all-encompassing discourse concerning mental health and illness.

Another obstacle to reaching some degree of clarity as to the nature of the debate was the multidimensionality of the polemics. There was an intrascientific dimension, where opposing schools of thought and opposing professional interests within psychiatry itself were voiced in seemingly irreconcilable terms. There was also an interscientific dimension: opposing views were adopted by philosophers, sociologists, historians, psychologists, physicians etc. And there was an extrascientific dimension where psychiatry was discussed within the contexts of politics, ideology and general debates on western culture.

A third complicating factor with regard to a penetrating characterization of the debate is the fact that the claims of the critics were raised at very diverging levels of ambition: psychiatry ought to be changed in this or that direction, psychiatry should be improved in this or that respect, psychiatry in its present form should be deconstructed and done away with, etc.

The aim of this study is not to attempt an encompassing analysis of, or to write the history of, the early debate on psychiatry.[2] The purpose is rather to return to, and reappraise, some of the central *arguments* of that debate. I shall, however, make a few suggestions as to important characteristics of the debate that have some bearing on the inquiries of this study. An important feature of the debate, I suggest, is that at the centre of most of the polemics concerning psychiatric issues, if penetrated with enough vigour, could be found a basic and fundamental issue: the dilemma of the concept of mental illness. The notion that a number of human and/or social problems could, and should, be conceptualized in terms of mental illness is central to almost every dimension of the debate; it is the common denominator and focal point of the questioning of psychiatry's scientific status and ambitions, of the questioning of psychiatry's treatment strategies and ideological platform, of the questioning of the legitimacy of psychiatry as an agency within the judicial system, and of a number of other issues raised in the debate.

My second suggestion is that through large parts of the complex and seemingly multi-faceted polemics on psychiatry-related issues runs a deep and severe opposition between two perspectives. We could call them a *medical-humanitarian* perspective and a *sociological-critical* one. Partly through focusing on different parts of the issues under debate, and partly through using very different analytical and interpretational schemes, adherents to the one of these perspectives tend to arrive at conclusions widely diverging from those of adherents to the other one, on most issues concerning psychiatric theory and practice. One way to achieve a sense of the contradictory and hard-to-reconcile characters of the two perspectives is to consider the very different ways in which the history of psychiatry, and the history of the coming into being of the medical-model conception of abnormal behaviour and mental afflictions, could be written. In the works of psychiatrists, like Redlich & Freedman,[3] or traditional historians of medicine, like Ackerknecht,[4] these histories are portrayed with a strong stressing of *similarities* between psychiatry and medicine in general. The roots of the medicalized view of insanity and irrational behaviour are sought, and usually found, far back in antiquity. The continuity of the historical development of psychiatric thinking is depicted as a matter of fact. Psychiatry is seen to evolve steadily through the centuries on the basis of scientific development and ever-increasing humanitarian efforts to find effective ways of curing human suffering and misery. Medical psychiatry is seen to fight bravely against superstition, moralism and prejudice, to eventually arrive at an established, accepted, enlightened and truly scientific view of insanity and other afflictions of the mind as diseases and appropriately medical problems.

If one turns to the writings of, for instance, Foucault[5] and Scull,[6] a totally different image of psychiatry will emerge. The driving forces, and "true" motives, behind the development of the psychiatric institution and the medicalized discourse on abnormal behaviour and mental afflictions are here strongly suggested to be extra-medical. Social, political and economic factors, connected to societal rather than individual needs, are shown to account for the establishing of psychiatry as a medical discipline and as an agency legitimized to intervene against individuals who, for various reasons, do not fit into the workings of modern society. The *differences* between psychiatry and "medicine proper" are stressed, and the lack of valid theories of "mental disease" and effective treatment-strategies, at the time when psychiatry was established as a medical sub-discipline, is highlighted.

The two perspectives really seem quite contradictory, and this divergence of views does not just stem from the focusing on different parts of the psychiatric-historical complex, but is to quite a substantial extent due to a divergence of interpretations of historical facts.

Closely connected to these two perspectives are the applications of two conceptual models to so-called mental-illness phenomena — a medical model and a sociological model. The distinction between these could be expressed in terms of two different and opposing ways to approach the question "How should we understand the term 'mental illness'?" I believe that most medical men, and most lay persons, would answer this question somewhat as follows: There is a category of human problems that we call illnesses. This category could be divided into two sub-classes: somatic illnesses and mental illnesses. The somatic illnesses concern the human body, and the mental illnesses concern the human psyche or mind.

This view, which seems almost ridiculously common-sensical and self-evident, actually contains the most central and controversial assumptions of the medical model of "mental-illness" phenomena: 1) that the phenomena called mental illnesses are sufficiently like the phenomena called "ordinary", or bodily, illnesses for the two categories to be subsumed under a common head-category, and 2) that the two types of phenomena are sufficiently dissimilar to motivate the separation of them into two distinguishable sub-categories. The espousing of the medical model, on the part of various participants in the debate, most often is tied to the notion that "mental illnesses are like any other illnesses"; they are entities or processes located within the ill person, causing suffering and incapacitation; and just like any other illnesses they could, and should, be diagnosed and treated by medical expertise.

The opposing view, pointing out the key features of the sociological model, of the term "mental illness" could be outlined roughly like this. What we have to take as our "raw material" of reality are different types of deviant behaviour. These are conventionally named "criminal behaviour", "prostitution", "drug abuse", etc. And among these sub-categories of deviance is a category called "mental illness". This category, named "mental illness" for historical and complex reasons (so goes the argument of adherents of this view), is the object of interest of a professional group and societal institution, psychiatry, that is the legitimized agency for dealing with the problems included in the category. But whether these phenomena are really illnesses, and what is to be meant by this, is highly questionable, and should be the object of close scrutiny. Along with the adhering to this model goes a denying that "mental illnesses are like any other illnesses". Adherents of the sociological model often make it their business exactly to show that "mental illnesses" are in important respects dissimilar to "any other illnesses", and that this provides the basis for refuting the medical-model conception.

Most of what I shall have to say throughout this study concerns the medical model. But it should be noted that an espousing of the sociological-critical perspective and the sociological model implicitly underpins much of the criticism of the medical-model conception of so-called mental-illness phenomena, put forward by Thomas Szasz and other critics to be discussed on the pages to follow.

When the early critics, often termed "the anti-psychiatrists", are referred to in recent literature on psychiatric issues, this is most often accompanied by severe denouncement. O'Connell[7] in a positive review of a 1986 volume entitled "The Reality of Mental Illness" by Roth and Kroll,[8] consisting of what purports to be a final rebuttal of the anti-psychiatric critique, asserts that there really ought not to be a need for such an enterprise any longer. The proposals put forward 20 years ago by Szasz, Laing, Foucault and Basaglia, questioning the notion of mental illness, should, he suggests, not really have to be addressed, since the debate has been settled: "Mental illness does indeed exist."[9] This attitude is somewhat typical of the way the early debate is quite often reflected in recent discussions of psychiatry. Apologists of psychiatry tend to claim that the attacks on psychiatry and psychiatric discourse were silenced by way of massive counter-criticism. The critics were refuted by sound and strong arguments in favour of the central theoretical premises on which psychiatric modes of thinking and acting exist, it is stated. "Today everyone knows that the critique was misdirected and flawed" is a rough characterization of this attitude. It is rarely, however, that this notion is supplemented with examples of any articulate reviewing of the nature of the critics' arguments or of the counter-critical arguments hinted at.

A quite different reason for abandoning the lines of critique adopted by the "anti-psychiatrists" is supplied by claimants to a more modern, updated and radical position with regard to the criticism of psychiatry. These, exemplified by Peter Miller,[10] tend to view the "anti-psychiatrists'" focusing on conceptual issues as oversimplified and passé. We should move from a limited conceptual discussion to a critique of psychiatry itself, its role in the larger context of the institutional settings of post-war, late-capitalist western society, and focus rather on the *doings* of psychiatry within a wide-ranging social and cultural analysis where conceptual matters play but a small part. With the overall intentions of these theorists I have no disagreement. The analysis of the emergence of Western late capitalist (or even post-capitalist) culture and social structure, where medicine (and psychiatry as medicine) should be analyzed as one piece of a giant jig-saw puzzle of social reality-construction, is a formidable project. I contend, however, that this project could not be successfully undertaken if the critique of the 60's and 70's was unfairly or incorrectly estimated.

Thus, contrary to these views of the early debate, I suggest that there are very good reasons for not letting "bygones be bygones", and on the contrary a case could be made for the necessity of returning to, revitalizing and reappraising some of the central arguments of the early discussion of the notion of mental illness. Briefly stated, three arguments could be supplied in favour of this suggestion. 1) Contrary to the implications of some apologists of psychiatry, there is no self-evidently correct assessment of the strengths of the early critique; there is no thorough analysis of the outcome of the debate. 2) The concept of mental illness, I contend, is the pivot around which the entire debate rotates, and without clear answers to the questions about the validity of this concept no really well-argued stand can be taken on issues concerning the scientific status, theoretical and practical legitimacy or "true" functions of psychiatry. The concept of mental illness, one could argue, after all is the *raison d'être* of psychiatry as a medico-scientific discipline. 3) There has occurred a substantial development of the philosophy and theory of medicine over the last 10-15 years, which makes a renewed testing of the strength of the theoretically oriented criticism of the notion of mental illness most interesting.

The central question

A matter that needs addressing in connection with this need of returning to the early debate on "mental illness" is the issue of the formulating of a question to be answered, with regard to the problems under debate. A necessary step towards developing a strategy for analyzing and assessing the strengths of various contributions, it would seem, is to formulate and pose a distinct, answerable question, that different lines of reasoning within the debate could be taken as attempts to provide arguments for an answer to. And this is no idle enterprise. "The technique or treatment of a problem begins with its first expression as a question", writes Susanne Langer, and "...The way a question is asked limits and disposes the ways in which any answer for it — right or wrong — may be given."[11] In the forms of the questions concerning a certain problem-area are hidden an attitude of mind and basic principles that govern and rule "the natural way of thinking" about the problem at hand. A number of questions, explicitly or implicitly asked in the debate on psychiatry and the mental-illness notion, seem less suited to provide the starting-point we need, since they would risk leading us astray or beg other, more fundamental, questions. I have in mind such questions as the following. "Are mentally ill people suffering?". "Are people suffering from mental illnesses actually quite normal?". "Is there a societal need for intervening against mental-illness problems?".

Two other suggestions for "the fundamental question" that would seem somewhat more reasonable must also be refuted. The first one is "Does mental illness exist?". This question is sometimes used polemically by apologists of psychiatry, in order to provide grounds for showing the absurdity of an answer in the negative, but it is built on a common misrepresentation and overstating of the claims of the serious critics. The problem of the notion of mental illness is not one of whether the phenomena called mental illnesses exist or not, but one of how these phenomena (that certainly do exist) should be characterized. The second suggestion to be refuted is this one: "How should a reasonable concept of mental illness be defined?". This formulation avoids, and understates, the thrust of the serious critique. This question is secondary to, and dependent on the answer to, a more fundamental question. The central question, I claim, is this one: "Is it correct to conceptualize certain abnormal behaviour and/or mental afflictions in terms of mental illness?". Or, more sharply: "Should there be a concept of mental illness?". This question is fairly equivalent to the following one: "Is the medical-model conception of abnormal behaviour and mental afflictions appropriate?". One advantage of these formulations is that they could (ideally) be answered with a Yes or with a No. Another advantage is that there should be little difficulty in separating Yes-spokesmen from No-spokesmen.

Aims and ambitions of this study

The aims of this study can be quite simply stated. The inquiry here to be undertaken aspires to reach an increased degree of clarity as to the strengths of some proposed arguments against the notion of mental illness or disease, and to attempt a problematizing of some suggestions of an elaborated defence of that notion. To suggest that the study should provide a definite answer to the central question would be over-ambitious as well as presumptuous. The issue under debate is a complex and intricate one and it needs thorough and careful analysis. Problematizing the current view that the medical-model conception of abnormal behaviour and mental afflictions is obviously unobjectionable, and that the critique of the 60's and 70's directed against that conception was misdirected and flawed, is in itself an important task, I contend. This aim could be viewed as part of a more far-reaching ambition to contribute to a revitalization of the discussion of the theoretical foundations of psychiatry — a revitalization that I believe to be urgent and important.

Some methodological preliminaries

A choice of platform and a distinction between two lines of reasoning

I shall make a choice of platform and "working-hypothesis" for the analyses by starting from the assumption that the critics — that is, the arguers for the "No"-answer to the central question — are in the right. Two brief motivations for this choice are the following. 1) The critics started the debate. Their arguments were formulated first. Not very much in the nature of explicit and strongly-argued defence of the concept of mental illness was really produced before the critique provoked such arguments. This makes the "logical order" of the exchange of arguments follow more naturally from giving the "No"-answer arguments the upper hand hand at the start of the investigation. 2) From a more personal and subjective point of view, I feel more comfortable with this choice of point of departure. My own primary intuitions led me to suspect, at my first aquaintance with the polemics in question, that there really is something problematic or unacceptable about the mental-illness concept. It goes without saying that this choice of working-hypothesis shall not be allowed to affect the critical analysis of reasonings and the weighing of pro- and contra-arguments in any biased way.

Having formulated the central question, "Should there be a concept of mental illness?" (or, equivalently, "Is the medical-model conception of abnormal behaviour/mental afflictions appropriate?"), I shall suggest that there are, distinguishable in the debate, two major lines of reasoning in favour of the "No"-answer. One aims at, through logical and semantical inquiry, showing that there is something inappropriate or confused about the concept of mental illness or disease in itself. This line of argument, that we could name philosophical, focuses its attention on the theoretical foundations of the medical-model conception of abnormal behaviour and mental afflictions. Another line of reasoning proposes to show that the functions of the mental-illness notion, on the level of individual, professional and societal interests, are in some way suspect, harmful or otherwise not to be wished for. This line of argument, that we could name ideological-critical, focuses mainly on an extra-theoretical, most often social or political, level of motives and arguments. The distinction is not perfectly clear-cut, since much arguing on the issue of the medical-model conception of abnormal behaviour and mental afflictions tends to combine and intertwine the two lines of argument, but I suggest that there are analytical purposes to be served by keeping it as clear as possible. It should be noticed that the arguments in favour of the medical-model conception could of course be distinguished analogously. Both lines of argument are concerned with conceptual issues, but in quite different ways. Most of what I shall have to say in this study concerns the more philosophical line of argument, but in the final chapter of the study I shall touch upon some ideological-critical points.

Some brief remarks are needed to counteract possible suggestions of a quite different way of reaching clarity on the issue of the concept of mental illness, viz. by way of empirical investigation. The appropriateness of a concept or a conceptual apparatus cannot be assessed by empirical means. Empirical science can verify or falsify statements, propositions, hypotheses, etc. If the content of the concept of mental illness had already been clarified and agreed upon, then you could go on to investigate empirically the reality of the phenomena included in the extension of the concept. Empirical investigation could provide answers to the question "Are the phenomena called mental illnesses caused by organic defects/traumatic childhood experiences/faulty learning processes/etc.?". But empirical investigations into the nature of "mental-illness" phenomena could not help us decide whether there should be a concept of mental illness or not. Suppose that empirical investigation were to tell us unequivocally that "mental illnesses" are due to organic malfunctioning (for instance some definitely localized CNS disturbance) or to psychological conflicts during childhood. This would not lead us one step closer to resolving the problem of whether or not the phenomena in question ought to be conceptualized in terms of mental illness, if we had not already reached an agreement as to the content of the concept of mental illness. If organic malfunctioning of the above-mentioned type was empirically found to be beyond any doubt the cause of some "mental-illness" phenomena, this would not at all self-evidently lead us to accept the notion of mental illness. It could perhaps direct us to build a case for rejecting it, since the phenomena in question would rather seem to be proper candidates for location in the extension of the concept of somatic illness. If the phenomena in question were shown to be explainable in terms of emotional conflicts deriving from childhood experience, this would only lead us to accept the concept of mental illness if we had agreed that illness could be defined in a way that allows for psychological disturbances to be included in the concept. Thus, much of the discussion of the concept of mental illness that claims to be founded on empirical research really seems to be missing the point. The question "Are the phenomena called mental illnesses correctly conceptualized in terms of mental illness?" could only be resolved by reference to empirical findings if a definition of illness and a definition of mental illness had already been agreed upon. Having stated this, which is intended as a retort to the possible objection that I do not deal adequately with empirical findings, and as a defence of the value and necessity of theoretical argument, I shall not direct my attention very much to empirical research on "mental illness" throughout this study.

Two postulates

The next step in this outline of strategies is to introduce two methodological postulates that will serve as basic underpinnings of my analyses and reasoning throughout the study. After the brief presentation of them below I shall take them for granted, and no further argument will be supplied in favour of them. The *first postulate* ("the comparison postulate") states that the feasibility (or non-feasibility) of conceptualizing certain forms of human behaviour and mental afflictions in terms of mental illness must be the outcome of a comparison of these "mental-illness" problems with "ordinary" or bodily illnesses. That is, it is through showing that the phenomena called mental illnesses are sufficiently alike bodily illnesses (or that they are not) that one can sustain (or refute) the reasonableness of the concept of mental illness. This implies accepting the notion that the concept of "ordinary" or bodily illness is the more basic, the paradigmatic and the far more well-entrenched concept. Support for this view could be drawn from a number of prominent defenders of the concept of mental illness, such as Boorse,[12] Macklin[13] and Margolis,[14] as well as from a number of outspoken critics of the concept, such as Szasz,[15] Flew[16] and Leifer.[17]

The *second postulate* ("the conceptual stringency postulate") states that it is desirable, worth-while and to some extent urgent to strive for conceptual stringency and clarity. This postulate, in one sense, constitutes a presupposition of the value and reasonableness of attempting an inquiry like the one here put forward. The postulate implies a refutation of such frequently encountered propositions as the following: "It is feasible to conceptualize a phenomenon however you choose to conceptualize it. It is what you do about it that is important!". "Concepts are constantly changing and developing and therefore it is futile to search for fixed definitions and to try to draw lines between proper and improper concept-applications.". "The 'true' meaning of this or that term could only be searched for within the framework of a realist philosophy that is no longer credible!". Contrary to this type of remark I shall contend that conceptual stringency and clarity is the ultimate goal of much worth-while scientific activity, philosophical and other, and that the striving for clarity as to the meaning of terms (both scientific and everyday ones), together with the pointing out of ambiguities, flawed logic and the rhetorical and ideological functions of the conceptual apparatuses of modern society, is not only legitimate, but ultimately what in many cases constitutes the hallmark of scientific critical activity.

The value of conceptual stringency is perhaps most readily recognizable if one considers the consequences of the lack of it. The mental-illness debate is an example of this, as good as any. Much arguing on the part of critics as well as apologists of psychiatry seems to miss the point, simply because key notions are used in diverse or too imprecise ways.

The recognition that conceptual clarity and precision of definition are ideal circumstances, sometimes extremely hard to achieve, constitutes no valid objection to this postulate. Accepting the postulate simply requires that one should regard a higher degree of conceptual stringency as preferable to a lower degree, and therefore worth striving for.

A note on the choice of Thomas Szasz's critique as a starting point

It is important to take note of the fact the grouping together of a number of critics under the heading "anti-psychiatrists" was a strategy on the part of the apologists of psychiatry rather than an outcome of self-proclaimed affinities among the critics in question, and almost every one of these critics has at some point renounced the notion of a common platform. The critics were actually a very heterogeneous group, differing widely as to ideological platform and motivation.

The reasons for my choosing the writings of Szasz rather than, say, those of the early R. D. Laing or David Cooper (with either of whom I feel more affiliaton on several points of value-orientation and political outlook), can be summarized as follows. Szasz's argumentation — and this of course is decisive — is far more stringently pursued. It is quite possible to make explicit the structure of his argument and to follow his line of reasoning (which is not, to my mind, always the case in the writings of Laing and Cooper). Very important is that Szasz's criticism of the psychiatric conceptual framework has provoked more counter-criticism than that of any other writer I know of, and it has to a quite unique extent forced apologists of psychiatric theory and practice to sharpen their arguments.

Notes

1 The use of the terms "illness" and "disease" is problematic for several reasons. Some writers use them as synonyms, while others make a distinction of meaning between them, and, among the latter, there is no general consensus as to how the distinction should be made. I shall choose to adopt the interchangeable (synonym) use in chapters 1-3 of this study, in accordance with the usage of most writers referred to in these chapters. (This goes also for the title of this study.) In chapters 4-5 various ways to distinguish between the notions of disease and illness will be seen to play a crucial role in the discussion.

2 Since the aim of this study is not to contribute to the writing of the history of the early debate on psychiatry, but rather to discuss some central arguments of that debate, I shall not attempt to provide an overview of various specific contributions to the debate. Reviews of major features of the debate are provided in, for instance, Miller, P.: Critiques of psychiatry and critical sociologies of madness, in Miller, P. and Rose, N. (eds.): *The Power of Psychiatry*, Cambridge, 1986, and in Conrad, P. and Schneider, J.W.: *The Medicalization of Deviance*, St. Louis, 1980.

3 Redlich, F. C. and Freedman, D. X.: *The Theory and Practice of Psychiatry*, New York, 1966.

4 Ackerknecht, E. H.: *A Short History of Medicine*, New York, 1968.

5 Foucault, M.: *Madness and Civilization - A History of Insanity In the Age of Reason*, London, 1967.

6 Scull, A. T.: *Museums of Madness: The Social Organization of Insanity in Nineteenth-Century England*, London, 1979.

7 O'Connell, R. A.: Psychiatry and Antipsychiatry, (a review of Roth, M. and Kroll, J.: The Reality of Mental Illness), in *American Journal of Psychiatry*, 145, 8, 1988, p. 1025.

8 Roth, M. and Kroll, J.: *The Reality of Mental Illness*, Cambridge, 1986.

9 O'Connell, R.A.: Psychiatry and Antipsychiatry, p. 1025.

10 Miller, P.: Critiques of psychiatry and critical sociologies of madness, in Miller, P. and Rose, N. (eds.): *The Power of Psychiatry*, Cambridge, 1986.

11 Langer, S.K.: *Philosophy in a New Key*, Cambridge, Massachusetts, 1976, p. 3.

12 Boorse, C.: On the Distinction between Disease and Illness, in Caplan, A. L., Engelhardt, H. T., Jr. and McCartney, J. J. (eds.): *Concepts of Health and Disease*, Reading, Massachusetts, 1981, and What a Theory of Mental Health Should Be, in *Journal for the Theory of Social Behaviour*, 6, 1976, pp. 61-84.

13 Macklin, R.: Mental Health and Mental Illness: Some Problems of Definition and Concept Formation, in Caplan, A. L., Engelhardt, H. T., Jr. and McCartney, J. J. (eds.): *Concepts of Health and Disease*, Reading, Massachusetts, 1981.

14 Margolis, J.:The Concept of Mental Illness: A Philosophical Examination, in Brody, B. A. and Engelhardt, H. T., Jr. (eds.): *Mental Illness: Law and Public Policy*, Dordrecht, 1980.

15 Szasz, T.: *The Myth of Mental Illness*, New York, 1974, (revised edition).

16 Flew, A.: *Crime or Disease*, London, 1975.

17 Leifer, R.: *In the Name of Mental Health. The Social Functions of Psychiatry*, New York, 1969.

2 The critical position of Thomas Szasz

Introductory remarks

The American psychiatrist Thomas Szasz has since the end of the 1950's in a great number of books and articles very intensively criticized the conceptual apparatus, the practices and the societal functions of psychiatry. His importance to the debate on psychiatry of the 1960's and 70's must be regarded as a major one, and few participants in the debate, whether they have counted themselves among the defenders of psychiatry or among its adversaries, have chosen to leave his argumentation out of account.

Szasz's work can be conceived of as an attempt to provide a well-argued "No"-answer to the central question of whether there should be a concept of mental illness. The arguments he supplies in favour of his contention that the concept should be abandoned are partly along the more philosophical line of reasoning and partly of the more ideological-critical kind. I shall focus almost entirely on the former kind of arguments in this study. My aim is to discuss some current objections to Szasz's criticism, with the intention of testing the possibilities of defending Szasz's position against those objections. The arguments of the opponents of Szasz will be discussed on the terms of those opponents. It is not uncommon, when Szasz's work is brought up for discussion, that his argument is presented in a very summary way, and sometimes it is also vulgarized and distorted. I shall therefore begin with a rather extensive and detailed and as accurate as possible overview of relevant parts of Szasz's criticism.

Szasz's criticism of the concept of mental illness

The criticism reviewed[1]

Thomas Szasz claims that "mental illness" is an improper word-combination. The term "mental illness", he suggests, is a deceptive metaphor that has become so thoroughly worked into our usage that we no longer seem to recognize that it connotes a concept that is self-contradictory, incorrect and misleading. There are no, and there have never been any, "mental illnesses". From this, it seems, follows also that psychiatry is incorrectly regarded as a medical sub-discipline; that psychiatric treatment is incorrectly regarded as medical treatment; that people who are treated by psychiatrists are incorrectly regarded as medical patients; and that the claims of psychiatry itself in these respects are groundless and should be rejected.

An analysis of the concept of mental illness, Szasz suggests, requires that the content of the concept of ordinary, or physical, illness be first elucidated. When we say of a person that he is ill we mean, according to Szasz, primarily two things: firstly that the person is believed to suffer from a physical abnormality or malfunctioning; and secondly that he wants, or accepts, to be a medical patient. "Illness" thus seems to refer on the one hand to some biological circumstance, and on the other to a social role.

This way of viewing illness, Szasz further suggests, reflects two fundamental premises underpinning the practice of Western medicine: that the physician's task is to diagnose and treat disturbances of the human body, and that he can do this only with the consent of the patient. This means that illness could really only pertain to the body. When we speak of mental illness we are therefore speaking metaphorically.

How and why, then, did the notion of mental illness develop? According to Szasz, up till the second half of the nineteenth century "disease" signified a physical disturbance, the typical manifestation of which was an abnormal change of the structure of the human body. "The Original Medical Game", Sasz proposes, had rules that made it possible to separate genuine disease (for instance when a person suffered or was incapacitated and this suffering or incapacitation was due to some abnormal change in his body) from that which just resembled, but was not really, disease (for instance when a person claimed to be suffering or incapacitated but this suffering or incapacitation was not due to any abnormal change in his body). This distinguishing of disease from non-disease also made it quite unproblematic to separate persons who were legitimate objects of medical intervention from those who were not.

But these rules were radically changed, Szasz contends, through the influence of Freud, Charcot and Janet. The dividing line between problems that were genuine diseases and problems that just looked like diseases was shifted so that some of the latter came to be included in the disease category. A conceptual change — a change of the criteria of what was to count as disease — accompanied and supported by a semantical change made it possible to speak of "mental" or "functional" illnesses as opposed to structural or organic ones.

Conversion hysteria became a prototype for this new class of illnesses, according to Szasz. The neurologist Charcot chose to emphasize the *similarities* (in terms of suffering and incapacitation) between the hysterical conditions and genuine diseases, and to neglect the importance of the *differences* (in terms of the absence of organic causes of the hysterical predicaments) which had up till then justified classifying hysteria as a non-disease. This choice, Szasz asserts, was not a matter of scientific deliberation, but was rather motivated by humanitarian efforts (on behalf of the suffering hysterics) and professionalistic ambitions (on behalf of psychiatry as an expanding medical enterprize). And he contends that this reclassifying of non-disease as disease was a definite mistake — a contention that some of his critics, as we shall see later on, takes issue with. Szasz takes great pains to elucidate the point that there can not be a meaningful concept of disease (class A) if we do not realize that there are phenomena that look like, but are really not, diseases (class B) and that there are also fake diseases (class B'). If we change the criteria, used for distinguishing between these classes, and let members of the latter classes become members of class A, the classification itself obviously becomes meaningless. But this, in Szasz's view, is exactly what has happened in medical psychiatry during the last 100 years. The concept of mental illness, he suggests, has made it possible to conceal the differences between two classes of human handicaps and problems: 1) physical diseases — disturbances in the human body viewed as a complex machinery — that could secondarily create social adjustment problems, and 2) problems of social adjustment that are not due to malfunctions of the "machinery", but rather to the purposes it has been made to serve.

In addition to hysteria Szasz points to schizophrenia as an example of how the dividing line between disease and non-disease was blurred. He states that Kraepelin brought together catatonia, hebephrenia and vesanica typica — three "conditions" that, however undesirable the behaviour associated with them, were not in themselves diseases — and claimed that they together constituted the disease dementia praecox. Bleuler then renamed the "disease" schizophrenia and widened the area of application of the term. Through the efforts of the pioneers of psychiatry an epistemological shift within medicine was accomplished: from histopathology to psychopathology. We should note, Szasz contends, the difference between the coming into being of these new "mental" diseases and the discovery of previously unknown physical diseases. Hysteria and schizophrenia were not made members of the class of diseases through the discovery of phenomena that satisfied the established criteria of belonging to the class if diseases. They were proclaimed to be diseases, despite the lack of any scientific discoveries that could justify this categorization. And, Szasz argues, this was made possible — as is the case with a number of behavioural deviations that during the last hundred years have been renamed mental illnesses — by way of a change of the criteria of what constitutes disease: from the presence of physico-chemical conditions of bodily disturbance to experienced, or imputed, suffering or malfunctioning.

The concept of illness, Szasz writes, points to deviation from some clearly defined norm, and in the case of physical illness this norm is the structural or functional integrity of the human body. Physical health, however desirable and positively valued, is quite possible to characterize objectively in anatomical or physiological terms, whereas the norm from which so-called mental illness deviates must be expressed in terms of psychosocial or ethical or legal concepts. It is obvious, Szasz claims, that psychiatric interventions very often are directed against moral, not medical, problems, and yet those interventions are supposed not to be subject to differences of opinion or ethical judgements.

When a person is suggested to be "mentally ill" this sometimes means that a disease of the brain is present, that accounts for the behaviour of the person. Biological psychiatry tends to hold that most (or all) problems denoted "mental illnesses" are of this type, and eagerly searches for the neurological defects that are supposed to correspond to this or that behavioural or cognitive disturbance. One then seems to suggest, Szasz points out, that "mental illnesses" differ from physical diseases only in that they are manifested in a different way — that is, by mental symptoms instead of by effects on organ systems. This, Szasz proposes, involves a mistake in that a symmetrical dualism is constructed between physical and mental symptoms. In cases of bodily disturbances in medical praxis you search for signs, like a fever, or symptoms, like a pain. But, he goes on, "mental symptoms" often refers to what a person has to say about himself or about his surroundings. He might for instance make suggestions about who he is or about his relations to this or that group of people. To regard those suggestions as symptoms requires that the person's beliefs and ways of looking at things are matched against those of the assessor or of the society they exist in. This shows, Szasz contends, that the notion of mental symptoms is not tied to a genetical and anatomical context, as is the case with the notion of bodily symptoms, but rather to an ethical and social one.

Szasz also takes into account that "mental illness" quite often seems to refer to some sort of deformation of an individual's personality, and that this deformation then is suggested to result in various difficulties and suffering when it comes to the person's meeting the demands of social life. He suggests that one has thereby made the implicit assumption that social life is by nature harmonious and that when it is disturbed this must be explained by illness, and he also argues that this way of reasoning means that "mental illness" has been turned into an abstraction that is supposed to cause certain types of behaviour and is no longer a description of those types of behaviour which it originally was.

An important difference between what is called mental illness and what is called physical illness is that the origin and phenomenology of the former are tied to claims or statements that people make, in a way that is quite different from what is the case with the latter, Szasz proposes. He points to the fact that physical illnesses could often be detected and diagnosed in routine examinations without any preceding claims having been made as to their presence, whereas diagnoses of "mental illness" are dependent on statements that a person makes about himself or that others make about him. In the absence of such statements or claims diagnoses of "mental illness" could not be made.

"Mental illness" thus really has to do with claims and justifications, rather than with disease and treatment, in Szasz's view and this, he suggests, also accounts for the fact that psychiatry has been tied up with law in a way that distinguishes it from the rest of medicine. The notion that "mental illness" sometimes causes certain criminal behaviour, and that the criminal in those cases is to be viewed as not responsible for his actions, has come to be uncritically accepted and made an important part of the judicial set-up. But since, according to Szasz, "mental illness" does not really at all signify any scientifically defined class of phenomena, the functions of the notion are not explanatory but rhetorical and justificatory.

What decides whether or not a person comes to be viewed as "mentally ill" or not, Szasz argues, is not what he does but what others think of his doings. "Mental illness" is a prescriptive term that is used as if it were descriptive and the use of it makes more difficult our understanding of the problems so denoted. The phenomena now referred to as mental illnesses should be removed from the category of diseases and should be viewed as "problems in living".

Some comments on Szasz's argument

Szasz's reasoning, on some points, gives rise to problems of interpretation. Most of those will be attended to in the context of the discussion of critical objections and counter-arguments in chapter 3. On some points, however, attempts at clarification would be pertinent before the commencement of that discussion. The question that Szasz's argumentation, at all times, is intended to supply an answer to, is this one: Do the many psychological problems and behavioural deviations that have come to be designated "mental illnesses" belong in the class of illnesses? Szasz argues for the answer "No". He does this primarily by way of pointing out what, according to him, are decisive differences between on the one hand "ordinary" illnesses — that is, physical illnesses — and on the other hand "mental illnesses". Some obscurities in his account then become prominent. An important part of his argument is the proposition that the kernel meaning of "illness" or "disease" is, or ought to be, expressed in terms of disturbance pertaining to the human body. He does not present an explicit definition that exactly specifies this kernel meaning. This seems to imply that Szasz himself bases his reasonings on an obscure concept of disease. The obscurity, however, is only partial. It pertains primarily to the problem of supplying criteria for distinguishing bodily abnormalities that are diseases from bodily abnormalities that are not diseases. This is of less importance to the discussion of the main issue. Szasz is after all, as we have seen, very outspoken when it comes to excluding non-physical disturbances from the category of diseases. The decisive demarcation line is thus drawn by way of stating a necessary condition of disease: the presence of physical disturbance. But then another obscurity of Szasz's reasoning becomes troublesome. The condition "presence of physical disturbance" could be interpreted in at least two ways. A strong interpretation, that sometimes seems to be the one intended by Szasz himself, is that demonstrable physical disturbance is a necessary condition of disease. Several of his opponents, as we shall see below, have pointed out that Szasz thereby seems to limit the class of diseases to including cases where the pathological mechanisms of a disease are known and clarified, and leaving everything else outside of the class. This limitation could reasonably be viewed as dubious.

A weaker interpretation is that a necessary condition of disease, according to Szasz, is that there is at least a reasonable *assumption* of the presence of physical disturbance. Some of Szasz's critics, for instance Macklin,[2] seem to prefer this interpretation. The condition would then admit that phenomena were classified as (physical) diseases even if the pathology were unknown; the meaning of "disease" would still be physical disturbance.

The choice of interpretation is of course decisive to an over-all assessment of Szasz's medical-philosophical reasoning, but the discussion of the main issue is also on this point affected only to a minor extent. Szasz's argumentation is primarily intended to show that "mental illnesses" — that is, problems and disturbances that are *not* supposed to be accountable for by physical disturbances — are not illnesses.

Szasz's criticism articulated in four theses

Before we turn to a discussion of objections to Szasz's criticism and an analysis of the strengths of those objections, it would be useful to attempt a summary of his view in the form of a number of propositions or theses, around which his argumentation against the existence of a concept of mental illness (as far as pertains to the part of his critique that has here been reviewed) could be said to revolve. I should like to formulate these as follows:

1) The coming into being of the concept of mental illness is associated with a mistaken extension of the concept of illness, that occurred through the efforts of Charcot, Freud and other pioneers of psychiatry.

2) The kernel meaning of "illness" is (or ought to be) physico-chemical disturbance of the human body, which is why you can only speak of "mental illness" in a metaphorical sense.

3) Ascriptions of illness in cases of physical and "mental" illness respectively are made on the basis of deliberations that are of very differing natures and that serve very different functions.

4) Human sufferings and troubles can be divided into two clearly separated classes: diseases, or illnesses, and "problems in living"; and the problems that are denoted "mental illnesses" belong in the latter, not in the former.

It should be noted that these four theses, or propositions, are interrelated in several ways, so that arguments in favour of, or against, one of them will often, directly or indirectly, constitute arguments for or against one or more of the others. The purpose of formulating them is primarily to provide some sort of structure for the discussion of a number of critical objections to Szasz's argumentation.

Notes

1 In the following summary review of Szasz's criticism I attempt to convey an accurate sense of the nature of his argument. The outline is compiled mainly from four of his works. Since my outline frequently wanders back and forth between major points of his argument in those four works I find it difficult to continuously supply the review with references in the text. Those parts of the review that concern the coming into being of the concept of mental illness are mainly drawn from *The Myth of Mental Illness*, New York, 1974, with the exception of the sections on the emergence of the concept of schizophrenia, which is founded on Schizophrenia: The Sacred Symbol of Psychiatry, in *British Journal of Psychiatry*, 129, 1976, pp. 308-316. The more general reasonings about the meaning of "illness" are drawn from The Myth of Mental Illness, in Scheff, T. (ed.): *Mental Illness and Social Processes*, New York, 1967, and from *The Myth of Mental Illness*, New York, 1974. The discussion about prescriptive and justificatory functions of the term mental illness is clearly elaborated in The Concept of Mental Illness: Explanation or Justification, in Caplan, A. L., Engelhardt, H. T., Jr. and McCartney, J. J. (eds.): *Concepts of Health and Disease*.

2 Macklin, R.: Mental Health and Mental Illness: Some Problems of Definition and Concept Formation.

3 A discussion of objections to Szasz's criticism

Introductory notes

The number of writers who have found it to be urgent to object to Szasz's criticism of the concept of mental illness could roughly be divided into two categories: those who claim that his criticism is absurd or unreasonable or imprudent, and those who claim that he is wrong and who supplement this contention with arguments. The attention will here be exclusively on the latter category. But yet another limitation is necessary, for reasons of space as well as of matter. Also in the latter category one can notice important differences as to the degree of willingness to interpret Szasz's propositions and arguments in a way that makes serious discussion possible and interesting. One reason for this is obviously an inclination on the part of Szasz towards polemical formulations and ironic commentaries. A good rule, however, is that you, if you are seriously interested in the issue under discussion, should prefer a more meaningful interpretation to a less meaningful one. What does Szasz mean, for instance, when he claims that there "are" no mental illnesses? A less meaningful way of interpreting this statement is to (like for instance Schoenfeld[1]) suggest that Szasz claims that the human problems called mental illnesses do not exist at all. This misinterpretation makes it possible to require (as Schoenfeld does) that Szasz should supply evidence that the persons that psychiatrists commonly treat are completely normal. But Szasz has not, to my knowledge, claimed that those persons are normal or problem-free, and no part of his argumentation is built on the premise that this is the case. What he does claim, emphatically, is that it is incorrect to interpret their problems in terms of disease, since the presence of problems and the lack of normality, in his view, are not, and ought not to be, sufficient criteria of disease.

The following presentation of, and discussion of, critical objections to Szasz will thus be limited to a number of objections that are built on meaningful and reasonable interpretations of Szasz's analysis.

On the coming into being of the concept of mental illness and the class of mental illnesses. (A discussion of objections to thesis 1.)

Szasz's claim that a mistaken or poorly motivated extension of the concept of illness occurred as a result of Charcot's, Freud's and others' efforts (thesis 1) could be seen as problematic from several points of view. One could argue that Szasz is right when he proposes that an enlargement of the illness-concept actually took place, but that he is wrong when he suggests that this change was illegitimate or that acceptable justifications were lacking; or one could argue that Szasz is wrong when he claims that an extension of the illness-concept occurred. Both of these objections are current among Szasz's critics. A third possible objection is more indirectly detectable among some writers: they imply that Szasz may be right on the matter of a conceptual enlargement having occurred, as well as on the matter of no strong reasons having been presented in favour of this enlargement at the time when it happened, but that we now, with the passing of time and events, could supply sound arguments that would make the conceptual extension, so to speak, retroactively legitimate.

Macklin[2] and Margolis[3] both seem to agree with Szasz's description of an extension of the concept of illness that made it possible to regard as illnesses certain problems that had not up till then been classified as such, but they reject his contention that this change was peculiar or wrongful.

When Szasz intends to account for his claim that an "error" was made, Macklin suggests, he sometimes construes the reclassification of psychological disorders as a conceptual or logical mistake, and at other times writes as if the change was "merely linguistic" or a matter of choice between differing classification systems from the point of view of scientific and practical usefulness. Szasz's position is therefore, she claims, unclear or even inconsistent. A strategy of counter-argument should, according to Macklin, have the following two stages: 1) showing that Freud and others were not making a conceptual or logical mistake when they started viewing psychological disorders as illnesses, but that they just performed an extension of the notion of disease or illness, and 2) showing that such an extension is legitimate — that is, that it can be justified by taking into account important and relevant similarities between cases of "mental illness" and cases of physical illness.

Macklin builds her argument, to some substantial extent, on the reasonings of Margolis, who claims that the extension of the concept of illness was legitimate as well as necessary, and that it does not obscure the differences between physical and "mental" illness, but that these, quite to the contrary, are preserved and respected in the very notion of enlarging the illness-concept. Such an enlargement of a concept could of course be justified, Margolis continues, through pointing out that new (mental) cases show such great similarities to old (physical) cases, that it seems reasonable to include the former into the concept of illness, and this was exactly what Freud and his psychiatrist colleagues succeeded in showing.

There are some problems that need addressing in this account. Macklin seems to imply that the conceptual change that Szasz criticizes could be conceived of as *either* a conceptual mistake *or* a conceptual extension, and that, if the latter is the correct interpretation, it only remains to show that the extension was legitimate, and Szasz's position stands refuted. This construction of the problem seems somewhat obscure. It is hard to see that a conceptual extension or enlargement could not be shown to *be* a conceptual mistake if it, for instance, is wrongful in the sense that it entails a change or confusion of the criteria something has to satisfy to be part of the original concept's extension. To be able to answer the question of whether or not the extending of a concept is a logical mistake, we must know what the original concept was like (its intension) as well as what the enlarged concept is like (its intension).

One should also, I suggest, apply some further criteria in assessing the legitimacy of extending the concept of illness or disease, besides the ones proposed by Macklin. It is important, of course, not just to observe the presence of relevant and important similarities between accepted instances of illness and new illness-candidates, but also to observe relevant and important differences. And it would seem reasonable to make an assessment as to whether it is similarities or differences that are more important and significant. One should perhaps also take into account the motives underpinning the enlargement of the concept, and make an assessment of them.

On the matter we are here discussing, Szasz's position could be said to be based on his contention that the differences were more important than the similarities when physical illnesses were compared with the psychological problems that were to be renamed mental illnesses. But the issue is not just one of making different choices as to whether it is differences or similarities that should be considered more important. Szasz claims, as we have seen, that there is a *fundamental* difference between physical illnesses or diseases and psychological disorders: in the case of the former, but not of the latter, we are dealing with organic disturbances. To look away from, or to underestimate the importance of, this difference involves, on Szasz's view, a definite mistake. The reason for this is that organic disturbance (according to Szasz) constituted the kernel element of what was then an established definition of illness. Or, to express this another way: if a necessary condition of disease (according to the original disease notion) is seen to have been dropped or obscured in the extending of the concept, it seems reasonable to claim that an error has been made from a conceptual point of view. Macklin's position would here have been a lot more clear if she had presented her views on the intension of the illness-concept before and after the enlargement of it. She suggests that it is not very obvious what criteria should apply even to the notion of physical disease, by way of referring to Margolis who suggests that bodily *symptoms* or *malfunctionings* (rather than, as Szasz suggests, bodily *causes*) should be viewed as the criteria of bodily illness. It is, however, as long as we are focusing on the question of whether or not a legitimate conceptual extension occured, important to keep distinct on the one hand the question of the correctness of Szasz's description of the established criteria of disease or illness at the time of the coming into being of the "mental illnesses", and on the other hand the question of which competing views on appropriate criteria of physical illness could be imagined to flourish after the changing of the concept of illness that made possible the illness-conception of psychological problems. To argue in favour of a "retroactive" legitimization of that conceptual change, on the basis of later changes in medical theory and practice, and in linguistic usage, is of course not unfeasible, but it seems inadequate as support of the thesis that the conceptual enlargement *was* legitimate when it occurred.

A benevolent interpretation of Macklin's and Margolis' arguments would be to take it that they suggest that there is a substantial lack of clarity pertaining to the meaning of "illness" before the discussed change took place (and that they claim Szasz's description in that respect to be flawed). If we adopt this interpretation, and if we conceive of Margolis' symptom- and function-based physical-illness criteria as current within medicine before one commenced to regard psychological problems as illnesses, the issue would seem to become somewhat different. We could then admit that an enlargement of the concept of illness that makes possible the existence of mental illnesses at least would not constitute *that* kind of mistake, that Szasz has proposed to be the case. This would however in no way imply that the conceptual enlargement was self-evidently legitimate. A central question (that we shall have reasons to return to later on) is if Margolis' physical-illness criteria should be thought of as completely detached from notions of bodily causes. Should this be the case it would seem difficult to make clear on what grounds a distinguishing of bodily from "mental" illnesses (like hysteria) could be performed (after the enlargement of the illness-concept). On the other hand, if some cause-related criterion after all is hidden in Margolis' suggestions as to how to characterize bodily illness (which on the benevolent interpretation would be supposed to be present before the enlargement of the illness-concept), Szasz's objections to the conceptual change would seem to regain some of their plausibility.

It should also be noted that even if Szasz's contention regarding the matter of the established meaning of "illness" before the arrival of Freud and Charcot should prove to be false, an assessment of the legitimacy of the concept-enlargement ought to include a consideration of the differences as well as of the similarities between physical illnesses and psychological disturbances.

Szasz's conception of the content of the illness-notion before the time of Charcot and Freud is, whether it is correct or not, a lot clearer than that of Macklin and Margolis. "Illness", according to him, unequivocally referred to a disturbance of the human body, viewed as a complex machine. Szasz's suggestions as to the content of the illness-concept after the enlargement of it constitute more of a problem. On the one hand he seems to propose that "illness" is a term that "really" continues to denote a bodily disturbance, but on the other hand he recognizes that a (however mistaken) conceptual enlargement has taken place.

A reasonable interpretation is that what Szasz is suggesting is that the meaning of "illness" all along has been, is, and should be, related to bodily disturbance. The change meant primarily that psychological disturbances began to be spoken of *as if* they were illnesses. There was thus seemingly an enlargment of the extension of the illness-concept — in the beginning, perhaps, with no intention of altering its content. This extension-enlargement, which entailed that "genuine" as well as "metaphorical" illnesses came to be included in the class of phenomena that were spoken of as illnesses, had as a consequence, according to Szasz, an obscuring of the differences between illness and non-illness. In that sense the change was primarily linguistic. When it comes to the matter of the intension of the illness-concept and any changes of this, the issue is more complicated. On the one hand we know that both Kraepelin and Bleuler believed "mental illnesses" to be physically caused. Similarly we know that one branch of psychiatry — that is, the biologically/biochemically oriented one — has sustained that belief up till the present time. On the other hand we know that a major part of psychiatric theorizing, from Freud onwards, is not built on that assumption.

What is central to Szasz's argument on this matter is that the criterion of bodily disturbance was dropped by psychiatrists of the latter persuasion, and that those of the former persuasion have all along been founding their ascriptions of illness, not on a study of the structure of the bodies of the patients, but on observation of behavioural deviations. Thus, he suggests, the two branches of psychiatry have mutually contributed to achieving the gradual shifting of focus from histopathology to psychopathology.

Pies[4] and Roth[5] both object to Szasz's claim that the meaning of "illness" that was established during the late 19th century included the notion of presence of a lesion. Pies proposes that ever since antiquity a dichotomy of views has existed within medicine. On the one hand there has been the view of disease as a specific lesion, and on the other the notion of disease as a phenomenon characterized by the patient's way of presentation. The latter, writes Pies, is not at all a view that developed as a result of the coming into being of psychiatry, and not even proponents of the former view, like for instance Virchow, suggested that lesions were the *sine qua non* of disease, even if they were assumed to constitute the basis of disease.

Roth proposes that Szasz has misinterpreted the process through which new diseases are discovered. It is not the case, like Szasz seems to believe, that medicine evolved through pathological changes first being discovered and illnesses thereafter being named. In most cases it is the other way around: a clinical description of a certain disease usually exists for a long time before its pathological basis is discovered. With Szasz's way of viewing matters Parkinsonism would not have been a disease from the time of the first description of it in the 18th century until just before World War I when the lesions causing the symptoms were discovered. The physical causes of diseases, Roth writes, had really been established in very few cases up till the last century.

Pies and Roth thus seem to unite in holding the view that Szasz is in the wrong when he claims that organic disturbance was a necessary condition of disease at the time before the emergence of psychiatry. They further seem to suggest, if I understand them correctly, that the "coming into being" of diseases like hysteria and schizophrenia was not associated with any change of the criteria of disease, but that the emergence of the "new" diseases could be described analogously to what is normally the case in the history of medicine.

If Pies and Roth provide a correct account, Szasz's position would seem to be weakened in several ways. An important part of his argument, as we have seen, is founded on the thesis that a criticizable change of the criteria of disease really took place, and his argumentation for a return to previously accepted criteria is, of course, founded on the assumption that these not only existed but that they furthermore were expressed roughly the way he describes them.

Certain objections to the position of Roth and Pies, as I perceive it, are however close at hand. Let us for the moment accept that a well-established notion of the meaning of "illness", based on what Pies describes as "the mode of presentation of the patient", and which supposedly would include experienced suffering and reduced functioning but not organic disturbance, was present well before the time of Freud and Charcot. The immediate question would then be: How should we explain that a number of psychological disorders not previously assigned to the class of illnesses were now in a relatively short time transferred to this class of illnesses? It would seem implausible that Charcot, Kraepelin or Freud *discovered* that many of those who now came to be classified as mentally ill experienced suffering and displayed reductions in functioning, and that no one had noticed this before. It could hardly be plausibly suggested that the entire volume of psychic and behavioural deviations that now were to be given psychiatric-diagnostic labels had not before the later parts of the 19th century been seen to involve misery and suffering on the part of the deviants themselves. Why, one must ask, is it that, if suffering and functional reductions were long-established criteria of disease, these problems had not far earlier been included in the category of illnesses? The fact that this had not happened (and on this matter there seems to be no disagreement) seems to strongly support the assumption that *some* sort of alteration of the criteria of illness really took place. It seems plausible to assume that the reason for these problems' not having been classified as illnesses earlier on, was that a distinction had been made between the kind of problems, sufferings and functional reductions that were due to disease and those that were not, and this distinction could hardly have been arrived at without applying some illness-criterion that excluded the latter. What might this criterion have been? A quite reasonable assumption would after all seem to be that this criterion had something to do with the presence of demonstrable organic disturbances, or with suppositions of such disturbances.

To deny that some conceptual change took place at all would seem implausible. Quite to the contrary one could suggest that if there is one point on which Szasz's analysis could find support from many directions, it would be precisely on the matter of the claim that a change took place that made possible the inclusion in the category of diseases of phenomena that had not previously been so included, and that this change was not due to some discovery, but that it required an alteration of the criteria of disease.

On the issue of Szasz's description of the ways new members of the class of illnesses "normally" emerge, the critics seem to indicate a weakness in his reasoning. Roth is of course in the right when he claims that in most cases a clinical description of a certain illness exists before its pathological mechanisms come to be clarified. The Parkinsonism example is striking, and if Szasz's position should be taken to imply that Parkinsonism did not "become" a disease until its pathology was clarified, it would seem strange. An important question here, however, is whether Roth contends that this example (and a number of others that could be given) just shows that Szasz provides a wrongful description of the way "new" physical diseases are discovered and included in the class of diseases, or whether he claims that the example also shows that the emergence of the "mental illnesses" is just as unproblematic and "natural" as the emergence of Parkinsonism and other "new" physical diseases. If the latter is the case, which seems probable since Roths's argumentation is intended to refute Szasz's thesis that the classification of psychological disturbances as diseases was a mistake, his reasoning would seem less successful. One could certainly argue that an important difference exists between the coming into being of "new" physical diseases and the coming into being of a new class of diseases, the "mental" ones. With regard to the former we are dealing with the identification of problems as diseases on the basis of important similarities to already established diseases. This identification does not require any alteration or amplification of the meaning of "disease" or "illness". The fact that one does not postpone the classifying of these problems as diseases until the pathological physical changes that cause the symptoms have been found does not necessarily imply that one does not assume the existence of such causes. On the contrary, it seems reasonable to imagine that the assumptions of the presence of such causes, the searching for them, and the belief that they will eventually be discovered, are important elements of the medical approach to the problems in question. When it comes to the emergence of the new class of illnesses, the "mental" ones, we are talking about problems with regard to which it is often not even suggested that there is an assumption of physical causation. In the case of Parkinsonism it was hardly suggested that there was being encountered a disease of a different nature from previously recognized physical diseases. On the contrary, it was, one would imagine, assumed to be a disease precisely on account of it being supposed to belong to the same category as that to which other, known, physical diseases belonged. Roth's Parkinsonism example therefore appears, if it is intended to point to the reasonableness of classifying (for instance) hysteria as a disease despite the absence of known organic causes, to direct us to stubbornly search for physical causes of the hysteric's symptoms. The same would go for schizophrenia and other so-called mental illnesses. His argument seems better suited for supporting the thesis that those problems are appropriate candidates for inclusion in the class of physical diseases than for underpinning the reasonableness of the coming into being of a new, and on crucial points very different, class of diseases.

An original, but somewhat difficult to understand, objection to Szasz's criticism of the "elevation" of hysteria to the status of disease is presented by Ross.[6] Ross suggests that Szasz's reasoning is somehow circular, and that he fails to recognize this on account of having subscribed so relentlessly to a notion of "illness" as identical with physical illness. If class A contains genuine illnesses, class B contains that which looks like and could be mistaken for illness without being illness, and class C contains deliberate imitations of illness, then hysteria, according to Szasz, from previously having been located in class C now came to be viewed as belonging to class A *and* class B. This implies, on Szasz's account, a classification mistake as well as a logical absurdity. But, Ross now suggests, this is a misrepresentation of the issue at hand. Class A contained physical illnesses. Hysteria, however, was not regarded as a physical illness but as a mental illness. That a phenomenon looks like physical illness, without being such an illness, and at the same time is an illness, does not constitute a logical absurdity if there is a superordinate species-concept of illness that contains the subordinate concepts of physical illness and mental illness. Hysteria was not proclaimed to be an instance of physical illness — indeed this would have implied a logical absurdity.

It is somewhat difficult to see what is thought to constitute the circular reasoning on Szasz's part. If we assume that Ross by circular reasoning means that one assumes what remains to be proven, it could be argued, however, that Ross himself comes dangerously close to such reasoning. There seem to be two suggested descriptions of the state of affairs, with regard to the existence of illness-concepts and illness-classifications at the time previous to the reclassification of hysteria as an illness:

1) A sub-division of the class of illnesses into physical illnesses and "mental illnesses" was already present and a super-ordinate concept of illness (which might then supposedly be thought of as defined in terms of functional reductions, suffering, etc.) was also present.

2) Such a division of illness into two distinct classes did not exist, and the concept of illness that was established was defined in terms of bodily disturbance.

Szasz presupposes the second alternative. His point is precisely that such a two-part division of illness as Ross speaks of was not established, and that this division on the contrary became established through, among other things, the "elevation" of hysteria to disease-status. The class of "mental illnesses" was created, on Szasz's account, through the efforts of Charcot,

Freud and other pioneers of psychiatry. And it is the creation of this new class that Szasz turns against, since he claims that no good reasons for the change in the concept of illness that was thereby necessitated could be presented.

It is more obscure whether Ross suggests that the first or the second alternative constitutes a correct description. It is apparent, however, that Ross views the classification of hysteria as illness as logically unobjectionable, and that he does not see it as a mistake precisely because hysteria was not included in the class of physical illnesses (which would have been logically absurd also on Ross's account). This seems to imply that he supports the first description. But if this is the case it appears strange that Ross neglects to make explicit that he views the basic premise of Szasz's reasoning (the premise, that is, that a change in the concept of illness and demarcation-line between illness and non-illness actually occurred) as false, which would make further discussion unnecessary. If Ross instead means that "the superordinate species-concept of illness" and the new class of "mental illnesses" did not exist previously but were brought into being through, among other things, Charcot's classification of hysteria as an illness, he seems himself, in his criticism of Szasz, to assume what remained to be proven. The reasonableness of classifying hysteria as an illness was supposed to consist in its classification as a "mental illness". But if the class of "mental illnesses" is created through the "elevation" of hysteria and other mental disturbances to the status of illnesses during the period in question, this "elevation" could of course not be *justified* by the existence of such a class.

A possible alternative interpretation of Ross's account is that he (like several other writers in this debate) slides back and forth between a discussion of conceptual and classificatory changes in the 19th century (whereby he aims to prove Szasz's criticism misguided) and a discussion of now accepted illness-concepts and -classifications (that he wants to sustain and defend).

The question of exactly how, and to what extent, the concept of illness or disease was changed during the 19th century is difficult to answer without a careful and thorough study of the history of medicine and the history of the philosophy of medicine.[7] We have seen that Szasz's opponents are in disagreement among themselves on this issue. That a change has occurred to the effect that during the second half of the 19th century and during the present century a growing number of phenomena not previously classified as diseases have come to be so classified, seems certain. It also appears obvious that the establishing of psychiatry as a medical scientific discipline is associated with the demarcation of a certain class of illnesses, the "mental" ones, and that within this class a great number of specific illnesses have been successively identified or constructed. It seems reasonable to agree with Szasz that the motives behind this medicalization of psychological and behavioural disturbances could not have derived from suddenly discovering that these disturbances were illnesses. The motives were probably of several kinds. That social-reform motives as well as medical-professional expansion-motives contributed as driving forces is probably a reasonable assumption. Whether or not these motives, in the light of the subsequent developments, should be viewed as justified is a complex question that will not be treated here. The interest here has primarily been directed towards trying out and discussing a number of objections to Szasz's thesis that the reclassification of psychological disturbances and behavioural deviations as illnesses was not scientifically well argued, and this has been performed on the terms of the writers supplying the objections.

It could be questioned whether this discussion of illness-concept changes and illness-classification reorientations during the 19th century is really interesting or important. The discussion should, it could be argued, be focused on such arguments for and against a medical conceptualization of mental afflictions and behavioural deviations as could now be supplied. One reason why the historical perspective is interesting, however, is that the platform of the discussion of the psychiatric illness-concept will be rather different if you claim that the notion of mental illness and the class of "mental illnesses" emerged through a questionable change in the concept of illness, as compared to if you claim that no such change in the illness-concept occurred. If you, like Szasz, suggest that such a conceptual change took place, you could argue that the burden of arguing in favour of this change rested with those who accomplished it — that is, with the representatives of psychiatry. And if Szasz is right when he claims that no sound argument was supplied, but that strong arguments against the change could have been presented, the change should be seen as a mistake. And this mistake persists, so to speak. It is just as wrong, on Szasz's account, to conceptualize psychological disturbances in medical terms today, as it was one hundred years ago. The burden of arguing in favour of this conceptualization therefore still rests with psychiatry itself, according to Szasz.

But from his opponents' point of view matters look different. Their positions when it comes to the historical analysis are somewhat divergent, as we have seen. But whether they suggest that no substantial change occurred in the concept of illness, or whether they suggest that such a change certainly occurred but was completely legitimate and correct, they seem to agree that today we have a concept of illness that in the first place is far more complex and wide than the one Szasz is pleading for, and in the second place could unobjectionably include the mental problems that Szasz would like to see excluded from the class of illnesses. From this point of view Szasz's criticism constitutes an argument for a narrowing of an established concept of illness, and the burden of the argument therefore seems to rest with him.

This divergence of opinion as to where the burden of argument rests would be worth keeping in mind as we now drop the historical perspective to embark upon a discussion of the meaning of "illness", and of what the significance of this meaning is to the existence of a concept of mental illness.

On differences and similarities between physical illnesses and psychological problems. (A discussion of objections to theses 2, 3 and 4.)

After what was said above about differences of opinion as to where the burden of argument rests in the discussion about the concept of mental illness, one apparently obvious objection to Szasz seems somewhat less plausible. Some of his critics (Ausubel,[8] Pies,[9] Roth[10]) suggest that in modern medical and everyday usage "illness" has a meaning that strongly deviates from the one Szasz proposes. It is pointed out that the concept of illness nowadays is multidimensional and complex, and that Szasz's attempt at narrowing down the meaning of the term "illness" is in strong disagreement with current usage. But referring to current usage in this case seems somewhat pointless, since it is precisely this usage that Szasz objects to and regards as wrongful and misleading. We should remember that the question under debate is one concerning what sound arguments could be put forward for and against the conceptualization of mental afflictions and behavioural abnormalities in terms of illness. It is therefore important not to confuse the factual presence of a medical conceptualization with the less obvious presence of strong argument in favour of it.

Common to many of Szasz's opponents is that they deny that the meaning of "illness" in any way includes the presence of organic disturbance, and that "mental illness" on that account would be an improper word-combination (thesis 2). The strategies employed to confront Szasz on this issue, however, are rarely founded on any particularly elaborate attempt at clarifying the meaning of the term "illness".

Roth[11] argues, by way of supplying a number of examples, that a sharp dividing line between that which is disease and that which is not could not be drawn on the basis of demonstrable physical lesions. A number of studies have shown, he suggests, that patients suffering from neuroses and affective disorders also very often show an abnormal amount of physical disorders. He also points out that the emotional disturbances that are typical in "non-organic psychiatrical problems" could be early manifestations of malignant diseases. There is a complex intertwining of personality factors, hereditary psychodynamical factors and physical handicaps that makes Szasz's drawing of the line impossible, he proposes. As regards schizophrenia it could be demonstrated that very similar syndromes have been found in cases of temporal lobe lesions; that in the case of older schizophrenics cerebral lesions have been found in a large minority; that certain chronic intoxications present a clinical picture that is very similar to paranoid schizophrenia, etc.

Roth's examples serve well to illustrate that there is a complex fabric of causal relations and affinities between various diseases, sufferings and problems. But it is hard to see that the examples could serve to support the thesis that the meaning of "illness" is, or ought to be, something very different from physical disturbance. Perhaps Roth's examples, or rather the fact that he produces them, could be seen as illustrating of the difficulty in dropping the notion of illness, or disease, as something related to the body.

Pies[12] takes issue with a suggestion of Szasz's that every physical disease that a person could "have", a corpse could also "have". A corpse could be said to "have" cancer, pneumonia etc., but to say that a corpse "has" schizophrenia, compulsive neurosis etc. would be absurd, according to Szasz. This, Pies suggests, is completely wrong. Virchow, for instance, that Szasz seems to view as a spokesman for the older and "proper" notion of disease, held that disease presupposes life and that disease as an entity disappears when the organism dies. If we thus assume (with Szasz) that it is a principle within pathology that lesions persist after the death of the organism, and assume (with Virchow) that the disease disappears at the death of the organism, we must conclude, Pies proposes, that disease could not be just the presence of a lesion.

It is somewhat difficult to understand what Pies hopes to attain with this reasoning. If his intention is to show that Szasz holds a mistaken notion of Virchow's view of whether or not a corpse could have a disease (or that Szasz and Virchow disagree on this point), he may have succeeded in this. It is doubtful, however, if Pies has here shown that disease is something that has nothing to do with lesions, which would be far more interesting. Certainly Szasz's position (that mental illness is an unreasonable or mistaken concept) is compatible with the view that illness or disease often implies the presence of a lesion plus something else. Pies' corpse-example is therefore unsuccessful if he intended to refute the proposition that the presence of a lesion, or the assumption of such presence, is a necessary condition of disease (of the body).

Pies furthermore seeks to show, by way of an example, that Szasz is wrong when he claims that physical illness is something that you *have* (whereas "mental illness" most often refers to what you *are* or *do* or *can do*, etc.). In cases of migraine the illness is often ascribed precisely on the basis of what the patient *is*, Pies suggests, (he *is* in a state of pain) and what he *does* (he *goes* to the doctor and *describes* his pain) and what he *can* and *can not do* (he *can not talk* when the pain starts, he *can not walk*, he *can not move*, etc.). When the doctor makes the diagnosis of migraine and prescribes a mixture of ergotamine, tartrate and caffeine, he does this precisely on the basis of those "is", "does", "can not", and not on the basis of a discovery of some lesion or pathophysiological change.

But once again the example appears badly chosen to serve as an argument against Szasz's thesis that disease or illness implies the presence of some abnormal physical change or the assumed presence of such a change. Why does the doctor prescribe a certain medication? He probably does not do this on account of this medication having supposedly positive effects on people's "being", "doing", and "being able to" in general. And why does he prescribe this precise mixture? The doctor probably does so because he holds a notion concerning a pathological change of an approximate type against which this therapy is supposed to be effective. What Pies does not seem to recognize is that in cases of physical illness the ascription of illness sometimes is made on the basis of what the patient "is", "does", etc. because this "being", "doing", etc. is seen as an expression of, or as caused by, a morbid physical change, whereas in cases of "mental illness" the ascription often is based on what someone "is" or "does" without any notion of morbid physical change being present (and often in the certainty that no such change is present).

Macklin,[13] as was referred to above, points to the factual presence of *different* classification systems and conceptualization approaches in the area under discussion. There is not, she suggests, any compelling evidence that it would be logically or scientifically incorrect to place emotional disturbances and psychological problems within the class of illnesses, rather than outside of it. What the arguer for the reasonableness of placing psychological problems in the class of illnesses has to show is only that the similarities between such problems and illnesses are sufficiently apparent to motivate such a classification. And this, Macklin proposes, has been convincingly shown by Margolis[14] and Ausubel.[15]

Both of these take as a starting point of their discussions Szasz's dichotomization of human problems into 1) illnesses — that is, malfunctionings in the human body, perceived as a complex machine, that could secondarily create problems of social adaptation, and 2) "problems in living" — that is, problems of social adaptation that are not due to malfunctionings of the machine, but to the purposes the machine has been made to serve by those who "built" it (parents, society) or by the one who "uses" it (the individual himself) (thesis 4). This dichotomization could not be maintained, they state. The dividing-line between disease and non-disease could not be drawn this way. And why could it not? The answer is that behavioural disturbances, emotional problems etc. on decisive points show such important similarities and conformities to physical diseases that many of them could well be included in the category of diseases.

Margolis thus proposes that psychogenic and sociogenic disturbances could be just as *incapacitating* as physical diseases, and could therefore in a reasonable way be conceptualized in terms of illness. We could in every instance of non-organic disturbance, and where the causes would be supposed to be mental, through a comparison with established examples of disease ascertain if the the similarities are substantial enough to make an illness-classification appropriate; and the aspect of comparison we should apply, according to Margolis, is the one concerning the degree of incapacitation or functional reduction. But is this an appropriate criterion of illness or disease? As we have seen, Margolis suggests that this criterion actually indicated the kernel meaning of "illness" even previous to the breakthrough of psychiatry as a medical discipline and the (on Szasz's view) therewith associated enlargement of the concept of illness.

Let us try the question: Should we perceive matters in such a way that *all* instances of insufficient ability or capacity-reduction that go beyond a certain limit are instances of illness? We should probably not. Functional reductions and capacity-limitations, as well as suffering, could be associated with, and caused by, a number of circumstances: poverty, starvation, ignorance, stupidity, oppression and persecution, sorrow and misery, deplorabe external circumstances of diverse kinds, etc. The main question here must be: How should we distinguish instances of reduced functioning, capacity-reduction and suffering that are instances of illness from ones that are not? It is difficult to see that the dividing line could be drawn (or could ever have been drawn) in a way that did not take into account the causes at hand.

Of course Margolis does not suggest that all human incapability should be interpreted in medical terms. He writes explicitly: "... medicine is an art of ministering to humans... in terms of *pertinent* incapacitation...".[16] But how do we decide which types of capacity-reductions are *pertinent* candidates for the class of illnesses? According to Margolis this question cannot be answered solely, or even primarily, in causal terms. What we need, instead, is a notion of the normal or characteristic or favoured forms of human life as regards capacity and incapacity. From this point of view, he proposes, insufficient or reduced capacity could be imagined to be due to any of a number of circumstances that would allow of explanation in medical terms — for instance, psychogenic and sociogenic circumstances.

But then we must ask: If it is the case that not all kinds of human capacity-limitation should be conceptualized in medical terms, but only the pertinent kinds, and this pertinence should not be primarily decided on the grounds of the causes of the capacity-limitations that are present, how could this medical conceptualization in a reasonable way be *motivated* and *legitimized*? It is difficult to see that the pertinence of the classification of diverse problems as medical problems, rather than as something else, should have nothing to do with the ability of medicine to describe, explain, and take measures to solve the problems in question. And it seems rather unlikely that the pertinence of this describing, explaining, and taking measures being performed within a medical frame of reference, rather than within some other frame of reference, would be to any substantial extent independent of a consideration of the causes of the problems.

Let us establish that nothing forces us to draw the line between illness and non-illness this or that way. The issue concerns what good reasons could be supplied in favour of this or that drawing of lines. When we choose criteria for drawing the line this or that way, we should reasonably do so on the basis of a notion of the criteria preferred being more appropriate than others from some point of view. It should not be denied that the criteria of illness proposed by Margolis indicate some important similarities between many instances of mental and emotional disturbances on the one hand and many instances of physical illness on the other. But the criteria would not help us draw a line between illnesses and a number of human problems that, according to accepted usage, are not illnesses, but that are all the same associated with suffering, incapacitation, etc. To achieve such a drawing of lines a substantial qualification and specification of the incapacitation and function-reduction criteria would be required. How such a qualification could be accomplished I shall not speculate upon in this context. But it should be noted that if it was to imply some form of discussion in causal terms, the strength of the argument in favour of an illness-classification of mental problems that is built on pointing to similarities between such problems and physical illnesses in terms of their *ef-*

fects, such as suffering and capacity-reduction, would probably be severely diminished.

A shortcoming in Margolis' proposal is that he neglects to answer the fundamental question of why we primarily, or a priori, should choose to point to similarities between psychological disturbances and physical illnesses, rather than differences. The same applies to Ausubel's argumentation. Ausubel suggests that an inclusion of mental problems and behavioural disturbances in the class of diseases could be made on the basis of the observation that the same essential *categories* of symptoms are present that are present in cases of physical disease. Diverse abnormal behavioural reactions to stress could be shown to be comparable to physical diseases in several relevant respects. Depressions and catastrophic impairment of self-esteem are thus, according to Ausubel, manifestations of personality disorder that is symptomologically comparable to edema in cardiac failure or murmurings from the heart in valvular disease. In both cases we are concerned with indications of underlying pathology in the form of inhibited functioning. He suggests that hypomanic overactivity and compulsive striving towards unrealistic goals are adaptive and compensatory responses to feelings of inadequacy, resemblant of cardiac hypertrophy in hypertensive heart disease or increased number of white blood cells in cases of acute infection. Distortive psychological defences, such as phobias and delusions, he points out, have some adjustive value but are generally maladaptive and are analogous to pathological situations in conditions like pneumonia, where the outpouring of serum and phagocytes is a defensive over-reaction that could cause the afflicted person to drown in his own body-fluids.

This pointing out of analogies between mental disturbances and physical diseases is of course plausible, but only if we have already made up our minds to regard and interpret mental problems as diseases. If we have not made up our minds to do this we should certainly ask: In what important respects do mental problems show *dissimilarities* to physical diseases? And how, and by means of what criteria, can we decide if similarities or dissimilarities are more important? And should we already, for some reason or other, have made up our minds to the effect that mental problems should not be conceptualized in terms of disease, it would surely be possible to point out categories of symptoms of physical disease that symptoms of mental disturbances would not fit into. The outcome of the comparison would be substantially ruled by what we were searching for.

The basic problem of Ausubel's comparisons, however, is that even if these behavioural or psychological reactions are clearly comparable to some of the symptom-categories that can be pointed out in cases of physical disease, it is doubtful whether the latter cases are spoken of as cases of disease on account of the presence of such adaptive, compensatory etc. reactions as are here in question. All of the bodily phenomena mentioned in Ausubel's examples are *reactions* to physical diseases. We are thus dealing with on the one hand an underlying pathology (for instance an acute infection) and on the other hand reactions to this pathology (for instance an increased number of white blood-cells). The question is then if Ausubel implies that the behavioural and mental reactions that he describes, in a similar way, are symptoms of an underlying psychopathological *cause*, and that this cause is the mental "disease entity". If this is not so, it becomes difficult to see why these mental or behavioural symptoms should be viewed as disease-symptoms.

It turns out, however, that Ausubel does not assume the presence of some such disease entity as a cause of the problems in question. On the contrary he claims that within psychopathology nowadays "mental disease" is not viewed as a cause of specific behavioural symptoms but as a generic term under which the symptoms are subsumed. This is important to Ausubel, since he does not just want to show that Szasz's dichotomization of diseases and problems in living is flawed, but wants also to vigorously refute Szasz's proposition that "mental illness" is a reified abstraction of roughly the same type as "witchery" or "possession". According to Szasz, notions of mental illness in terms of "deformed personality" and the like would function as supposed explanations of behavioural disturbances in psychiatric theorizing. Since one, still according to Szasz, cannot produce any plausible description of these internal pathological changes, the disease notions become almost demonological in character. But Ausubel claims that Szasz on this point provides an incorrect representation of what is meant by "mental disease". This disease is thus, according to Ausubel, in modern psychopathology not supposed to be constituted by some cause, inherent in the individual, that explains behavioural symptoms.

But if Ausubel is right on this point it becomes obscure how the analogy between behavioural symptoms and physical-disease symptoms could be used to support the notion that we are dealing with diseases in both cases. Heart-murmurings, excessive number of white blood-cells and excessive out-pouring of serum were to serve as examples of *disease-symptoms* in cases of underlying diseases (valvular disease, acute infection, and pneumonia). Of *what*, then, are the corresponding behavioural symptoms — depression, hypomanic overactivity and phobias — symptoms? If they are symptoms of something other than underlying pathological changes, why should we view them as disease-symptoms?

Let us here make a brief detour from the discussion of Ausubel's symptom-category comparisons, and attempt problematizing his proposition that modern psychiatry does not work on the assumption of "mental disease" as a cause of behavioural symptoms, inherent in the individual, but that "mental disease" is just a generic term under which those symptoms are subsumed. A statement to the same effect is made by Moore,[17] and Macklin[18] quotes Redlich and Freedman[19] who hold the same view.

The proposition appears strange from several points of view. If "mental disease", or "illness", is just a description of certain behaviours we would 1) have no possibility of explaining the behaviours in question by referring to the "mental illness", 2) have no possibility of distinguishing cases where a certain behaviour would be viewed as accountable for by "mental illness" from cases where a similar behaviour would be viewed as accountable for by something else, and 3) have no possibility of distinguishing "genuine" illness behaviour from simulated illness behaviour.

Generally speaking we consider it, on most occasions, possible to distinguish between different explanations of a deviant behaviour. Suppose that the following information is given about a person, P, unknown to us. P behaves in a seemingly extremely irrational way. P's speech is incoherent, illogical and difficult to understand. P makes, seriously and intentionally, obviously absurd and incorrect statements about himself and about the reality surrounding him, and when this is pointed out to him P stubbornly holds on to his statements and seems furthermore sometimes not to understand the objections. Now, suppose that one, on the basis of this information and while awaiting further details, forms the preliminary hypothesis that P is "mentally ill". The question is: When this assumption is made, does "mental illness" refer to the described behaviour or to the causes of the behaviour? Suppose that additional information regarding P were to be supplied. The information consists of the statement 1) that P is a three-year-old child, or 2) that P is heavily drunk, or 3) that P suffers from severe brain damage as a consequence of repeated haemorrhages of the brain. It is probable that one on the basis of this additional information would abandon the hypothesis that P is "mentally ill". One would drop this hypothesis, not on account of the description of P's behaviour having been proved incorrect, but on account of a cause, explaining P's behaviour, now being known, and this cause being something other than "mental illness".

With regard to a person's young age, a person's state of drunkenness, and a person's lack of cerebro-physiological integrity, these are matters that could, in principle, be established without making the detour of deduction from his behaviour. Is this what Ausubel and others are implying when they state that modern psychiatry does not view "mental illness" as an "entity" that causes symptoms in the shape of behavioural deviations? Are they saying that we could not arrive at a substantial cause, in this case "mental illness", of a behaviour the same way that we can point to for instance a high percentage of alcohol in the blood as a cause of a behaviour? But we have just seen that "mental illness" could not be only a description of a behaviour. It is hard to entirely escape the slight suspicion that Ausubel and others suggest that we apply "mental illness" as a descriptive term when we cannot find a plausible explanation of a (deviant) behaviour. But if this should be the case the term "mental illness" would really appear dubious. It would then seem to work primarily as a sort of fictitious explanation or pseudo-explanation, the main purpose of which would be to allow us to express descriptive (and pseudo-explanatory) statements on behaviours that we could not explain. With this interpretation it is difficult to see in what respects the term "mental illness" is more appropriate or well-functioning than "possession", "witchery", or "hocus-pocus". I believe that we with a high degree of probability can draw the conclusion that Ausubel and others are wrong when they claim that "mental illness" is a term the meaning of which has no association with notions of causes that could be more or less reasonably described. The theoretical ambitions of modern psychiatry are certainly far greater than they assume.

Let us, however, turn our attention away from Ausubel's and others' problematic reasonings in this respect, and for a moment imagine that we really are dealing with mental "disease-entities" that cause diverse behavioural symptoms. Could Ausubel's symptom-category analogies then be regarded as arguments for viewing mental disturbances as diseases? I believe they could not. It is apparent that the disease-symptom character of the physical reactions that he mentions is not at all primarily dependent on their adaptive, compensatory etc. characteristics, but on the fact that they are causally related to an underlying pathology. Heartmurmur that is not related to any underlying pathological disturbance would, if it were to occur, certainly be abnormal, but it would not be a disease-symptom. To make the analogy useful to support the view of the mentioned behavioural reactions as disease-symptoms, Ausubel would have to show what is the underlying pathology in those cases (and in what sense it is pathological).

Neither Margolis' separate-cases comparisons nor Ausubel's symptom-category analogies provide us with any theoretically compelling reasons for incorporating emotional disturbances or behavioural deviations into the class of illnesses. This would, however, not necessarily prevent us from regarding such comparisons and analogies as supportive of such a classification if we had already, for some or other reason, decided that such a classification were appropriate or to be wished for. What would such a reason be? One possibility would of course be to take seriously Margolis' description of medicine as an enterprise that aims at helping people who suffer from capacity-reductions of the "pertinent" kind, and to let the pertinence be decided on the basis of the demonstrated *competence* of medicine in this respect. Perhaps it is the case that medicine simply has proven to be exceptionally proficient and successful in solving diverse problems concerning mental and behavioural disturbances? Many would undoubtedly argue that this is the case. Others would argue the opposite. Who is right will not be discussed in this context. It should be noted, however, that a classification of mental problems as illnesses on such grounds would seem to be somewhat ad-hoc-inclined. The mental problems would be suitable candidates for such classification for purely pragmatic reasons, more specifically because medicine (that is, psychiatry as a medical subdiscipline) had proven able to solve them. And if, in the future, other (non-medical) measures were to prove more adequate, would the problems in question then, as a logical consequence, stop being medical problems? To argue for the reasonableness of this contention would be to risk undermining the basis of psychiatry's identity as a medical subdiscipline. It seems reasonable to assume that the proponents of psychiatry in general would hold that psychiatry as a theoretical and practical medical discipline is concerned with a category of human problems because it is proposed that those problems *are* medical problems, and not the other way around; that is, that the problems in question must be named illnesses because psychiatry on the one hand is effective in solving them, and on the other is eager to be called a medical discipline. Or, in other words, it seems reasonable to assume that psychiatry also claims to be able to theoretically justify its being regarded as having the character of a medical science and practice.

Moore[20] proposes, in accordance with Ausubel and Margolis, that Szasz is wrong in suggesting that "illness" ordinarily refers to some abnormity of the body (thesis 2). "Illness" was a word in the English language a long time before anyone knew anything of anatomy or physiology. The meaning of "illness" could therefore not be tied to notions of deviation from statistical physiological or anatomical norms, he writes. We have already encountered this argument. Let me briefly state the two objections that are most close at hand: 1) It could be argued to be of little relevance to our present discussion what meaning "illness" had two hundred or four hundred or fifteen hundred years ago. To deny the development of knowledge of medical science any influence on the connotation of the term "illness" would seem awkward. 2) The meaning of "illness" could well be thought to be deviation from biological normality even if knowledge of the more precise nature of the deviation were lacking in the individual case.

To be ill, Moore suggests, seems to imply "...something like being in a state of pain or discomfort, which, if not removed, may lead to premature death, and which, for its duration, incapacitates the patient from certain activities thought normal in our society."[21] And he suggests that although one might assume that such states have physical causes, this is irrelevant to what we mean by "illness".

But are such assumptions irrelevant? Is there no possibility of distinguishing such states of pain, incapacity and threat of death as are due to illness from such that are not? Suppose that I, by some malevolent person, am tied to my chair in such a way that I 1) am caused persistent and severe pain, 2) cannot move, and 3) have the normal blood-supply to vital organs seriously inhibited. Or suppose that I, on account of a misunderstanding, come to hold the notion that I am suffering from a life-threatening disease and that any mental or physical strain could be fatal; my false notion of my state of health keeps me in bed in a condition of deep anxiety, depression and inability to act. Am I ill (in the ordinary sense of the word) in either of these cases? I believe it would be to severely violate our usage to claim that this is the case.

The examples might seem far-fetched, but at least they show two things: 1) that "illness" reasonably would be seen to demarcate a subclass within the class of "states of suffering and reduced capacity", and 2) that this subclass could hardly be demarcated any other way than with the aid of some cause-related criterion.

Moore further states that concepts of *particular* illnesses — polio, pneumonia, etc. — include knowledge of physical causes, but whether or not someone is ill (in general) is not determined by the presence of such causes. Therefore it was correct to call for instance hysterics ill, he suggests. But could you really be ill without suffering from, or at least being supposed to suffer from, an illness? Could you be a hysteric without having the illness of hysteria? And if this is the case, then in what sense is this "illness" a medical problem? Do we ever, except in the case of "mental illnesses", claim that someone "is ill" if we do not at least suspect his "illness" to be accountable for by a physico-chemical abnormality, though perhaps of an unknown or just vaguely imagined nature?

Let me recapitulate what the issue that we are discussing is all about. Szasz has claimed that the difference between two classes of human problems, illnesses and "problems in living", should justify that the dividing line between them be kept clear, and that what is called "mental illness" belongs in the latter class (thesis 4). An important reason for this is, according to Szasz, that the meaning of "illness" is the presence of some biological circumstance constituting a disturbance of the human body viewed as a complex machinery (thesis 2). The objections to this position involve demonstrating that the similarities between certain mental problems and physical illnesses are substantial, and that the kernel meaning of "illness" is not associated with any notion of physical abnormality. The arguments in favour of these objections often imply that it could be shown that "illness" primarily refers to suffering, incapacitation and functional reduction, but that the notion of physical causation is not part of the meaning of "illness". We have seen, however, that this argumentation is associated with certain problems, and that it must be qualified in several respects if it is to serve as support for the view that psychological problems could unobjectionably be conceptualized in terms of illness.

Let me attempt yet another problematizing of the relevance of this argumentation to the issue under discussion by posing the question: Is this that is called mental illness always associated with suffering and incapacitation? With regard to the use of the term "mentally ill" it could be meaningful to make a distinction between two ways to use it: 1) "mentally ill" as a designation of persons who themselves claim to be suffering or incapacitated (and where no physical disease could be demonstrated), and 2) "mentally ill" as a designation of persons who behave in a way that is perceived by others as strange, threatening, disturbing, etc. (and where the causes are taken to be disturbances of the mind of the person) but where the person himself does not claim to experience suffering or incapacitation. If the meaning of "illness" is suffering and incapacitation — as Margolis, Ausubel, Moore, and others suggest when they want to argue for the reasonableness of placing mental problems or disturbances in the category of illnesses — we seem to face this choice with regard to the persons of whom the term "mentally ill" is used in the second of the above-mentioned ways: either we establish that these persons do not satisfy the criteria for being regarded as ill, or we suggest that these persons are not conscious of their suffering and their incapacitation.

The latter alternative probably has many proponents. A common suggestion about persons who are designated "mentally ill", especially in the case of psychoses, is that they lack awareness of their illness. This lack of awareness of one's illness could then be conceived of as consisting in the ill person's not realizing that he suffers and/or is incapacitated. Let us, in this context, leave out of account the substantial problems that would seem to be associated with clarifying what this *means*. We shall here just turn our attention to the question of what Moore, and others, imply when they state that a central criterion of illness is that suffering, reduced functioning and incapacitation are really at hand. When they propose that we normally — that is, in typical cases of physical illness — use the term to refer to the presence of those circumstances, do they then mean to say that in those cases it is the ill person himself who experiences suffering, incapacitation etc., or do they mean to say something else? If the former is what is intended, we must conclude that the criterion of illness is not satisfied in the instances of "mental illness" that we are now considering. If they mean to say something else, whatever this might be, we should remember that this something has to apply to physically ill persons *and* "mentally ill" persons if the meaning of "illness" is to be demonstrated to be identical in the two categories. Suppose for instance that the intended meaning is that it is such presence of suffering and incapacitation in a person as is established by one or more *other* persons, that is the criterion of illness (but that it is beside the point what the thus assessed person himself has to say). We must then ask: Does that kind of situation in fact ever occur in instances of physical illness? Even if such cases were to be shown to exist, we would have to state that they are not at all typical cases of physical illness. And in any case the similarity between mental problems and physical illnesses that is assumed to justify the classification of the former as illnesses ought, one could argue, to be a similarity between instances of mental or behavioural problems and precisely *typical* instances of physical illness.

To apply the term "mental illness" to persons who do not regard themselves as suffering or incapacitated is thus associated with some problems, if one simultaneously suggests that the meaning of "illness" is suffering and incapacitation. One possibility is now of course to suggest that we in the discussed cases of "mental illness" are dealing with a separate meaning of "illness". But then it remains to be demonstrated what is the separate justification and argument that would convince us of the reasonableness of this separate meaning. The arguments referred to up to now would then be of little relevance.

Apart from attempting to show that the meaning of "illness" is such that mental and behavioural problems could be appropriately classified as illnesses, Moore takes issue with Szasz's suggestion that a psyche, or mind, is not such an entity as can be meaningfully spoken of as "ill" or "diseased" or "sick". The difficulty with regard to answering the question, "What is a sick mind?", Moore proposes, is mainly due to the difficulty with regard to saying something intelligent about what a mind is at all. We could however, he suggests, leave this question, and instead ask ourselves: Has "mental illness" got as significant a descriptive and/or explanatory use as other expressions containing the word mental? And Moore proposes to be able to show that this is so. We use the expression "mental illness" to deny that the action/intention predicates can be as regularly and properly applied to the "mentally ill" as they can to the mentally normal, he states. We use the term to express that the behaviour of the person in question is not rational, and that we cannot use the form of description/explanation of his behaviour that we ordinarily use to understand ourselves or each other in everyday life. And thereby we could also express what a "sick mind" is, Moore writes. It is an incapacity to act rationally. "To say that someones' mind is ill is only to say that his capacity for rational action is diminished, that the subject himself is irrational."[22] Moore's discussion is here founded on a thorough and clarifying analysis of what we ordinarily mean by rationality. This analysis, that there is no ground for questioning the reasonableness of, I shall not review since it is in my opinion irrelevant to the issue under discussion. The main objection to Moore must of course be that his reasoning is only interesting and relevant if it has already been shown (for instance by way of a qualified and unobjectionable analysis of the meaning of "illness") that mental problems should be classified as illnesses. The most relevant question is *not*, "Has 'mental illness' as significant a descriptive/explanatory use as other expressions containing the word 'mental'?". It is instead, "Has 'mental illness' as significant a descriptive/explanatory use as 'physical illness'?" And this question could not be answered in the absence of a well-argued position as to what is to be meant by "illness".

To propose that the person's mind or psyche is ill, whose capacity to act rationally is diminished, does not seem very enlightening. It is difficult to see what additional information we bring to a proposition of irrationality on the part of a person by proposing that the person is "mentally ill", if "mentally ill" is the same as "irrational". I cannot see that Moore could be understood any other way than as suggesting that "mental illness" is just another *name* for reduced capacity for rational behaviour. But if this is the case, we should ask: Is all irrationality the same as "mental illness"? Have we got no way of distinguishing between irrationality that is supposed to be due to "mental illness" and irrationality that is accountable for by other circumstances? And should it be possible to imagine irrationality to be due to circumstances other than "mental illness" (such as stupidity, ignorance, or the uncritical acceptance of irrational collective beliefs) then how would we distinguish the sub-category of irrationality that is, or is due to, "mental illness" from other sub-categories? To be able to do this we shall of course require some criterion other than the irrationality itself.

To the discussion of Moore's reasoning could furthermore be added the observation that he, in accordance with several others who discuss "mental illness" in terms of irrationality, seems to neglect to make a clear distinction between "insanity" and "mental illness". That "insane" (or "mad" or "crazy") is an epithet which we in everyday language often attach to a person who behaves in a seemingly irrational way (or which we, alternatively, attach to the irrational behaviour itself), especially if we cannot find some plausible explanation of his irrationality, is probably correct. But the terms "insanity" and "mental illness" are not self-evidently synonymous. Moore, in his reasoning about diminished rationality, uses the term "mental illness" when he should plausibly use the tern insanity. That insanity is the same as, or due to, "mental illness", should not be presupposed without question. This is after all, one could argue, what Szasz objects to, and precisely what his critics need to demonstrate.

So far the discussion has been focused primarily on the critical objections to Szasz's illness/problems-in-living dichotomy that seek to demonstrate similarities between the two categories. Quite a few objections are also founded on attempts to refute Szasz's suggestions of important dissimilarities. Let us, in the following, turn our attention primarily to Szasz's propositions about differences in ascriptions of physical illness and "mental illness", respectively (thesis 3). Particularly problematic, he states, is that the concept of mental illness is used as if it were descriptive, whereas it is actually prescriptive, and that it is used as if it were explanatory, although it is in fact justificatory.

Brody[23] objects, on this point, that Szasz's account is confusing, since he sometimes claims that the concept of mental illness is mistakenly used as if it was descriptive, and sometimes that it is mistakenly used as if it was explanatory. But in general a description is not equivalent to an explanation. Brody therefore chooses to rewrite in the following way the thesis he would like to argue against: "The current use of concepts of mental illness creates difficulties because it uses a prescriptive concept (one used to justify certain behaviour towards people) as though it described or explained the behaviour and state of the people in question."[24]

Szasz suggests that diagnoses of "mental illness" are founded on claims that the patient makes about himself, or that others make about him, whereas diagnoses of physical illnesses do not have to be based on such claims. But this is simply wrong, Brody writes. In diagnosing "mental illnesses" you could very well utilize observations of behaviour that could be observed and verified. Szasz has suggested homosexuality as an example of a claim-based diagnosis, but homosexual behaviour could, according to Brody, certainly be observed and registered whithout any claims being made by the homosexual himself or by someone else. Claims are thus not the basis of the diagnosis, but should rather be viewed as additional behavioural evidence that could be utilized in the making of the diagnosis together with other behavioural evidence.

Furthermore it seems, Brody proposes, that Szasz also suggests that diagnoses in cases of "mental illness" are only guesses or conjectures. The doctor cannot know for sure if a woman is frigid or not. He can only make conjectures. But this also often applies to diagnoses of bodily illnesses, Brody writes. And suppose that diagnoses of "mental illnesses" really were claim-based; why would we from this conclude that such diagnoses are prescriptive, justificatory claims disguised as descriptive and explanatory claims?

Brody here seems to neglect, or discount the importance of, a number of factual differences as to the significance of claims in diagnoses of physical and "mental"illnesses, respectively. It is certainly correct that diagnoses of "mental illnesses" are often based on a combination of direct behaviour-observations and claims made by the patient himself or by someone else. But the interesting point here is that claims often are sufficient as a basis of psychiatric diagnoses, or sometimes really are the only possible basis of such diagnoses, whereas diagnoses of physical illness are rarely based only on claims. Furthermore it is obvious that claims in diagnoses of physical illness very often can be verified in a totally different way than claims in cases of "mental illness". A claim of pain, nausea, itching, paralysis, etc. could be made the basis of a diagnosis of physical illness if a physical examination showed that such an illness was present as probably caused these symptoms. In "mental illness" there is no such physical cause that could be detected and verify the claim. Therefore the diagnosis will often be based on what the patient proposes about himself or what others propose about him. "I hear voices", "I have visions", "I am sexually attracted to persons of my own sex" are claims that would be difficult to verify the same way that claims like "I have stomach pains", "I cannot lift my right arm", etc. could be verified. Moreover it is of course the case that a psychiatrist who is faced with the claim "I am a homosexual" does not really perform an observation of the patient's behaviour in the relevant respect, but will take the claim as a piece of information concerning what the patient feels and experiences and make his diagnosis on the basis of this.

Brody also suggests that even if claims about "mental illness" are conjectures, it does not follow that they could not be correct conjectures of what really explains a behaviour. You could weigh and evaluate whether guesses as to the causes of behaviours were either more or less credible by observing whether there was behavioural evidence to support them. This procedure is not at all different from the search for causes within the natural sciences. It seems, Brody writes, as if Szasz has not understood the basic epistemological relation between people's behaviour and our hypotheses of their mental lives, the healthy as well the ill.

Again one could argue that Brody here seems to neglect what could be suggested to be the point of Szasz's reasoning. Substantial differences between the "qualities" of conjectures and hypotheses of causes in cases of physical and "mental illness", respectively, could be pointed out. It could also be suggested that the claims to explain something with the aid of those conjectures and hypotheses are often enough more well-founded when it comes to physical illness than when it comes to "mental illness". Szasz proposes that diagnoses of "mental illnesses" only appear to explain behaviours, but really only put labels on them and point to and justify a measure. Objections to this proposition should reasonably be underpinned by arguments for the explanatory value of psychiatric diagnoses being acceptable, rather than by pointing out the circumstance that explanations in diagnoses of physical illness may sometimes be uncertain.

Brody also turns against Szasz's claim that there is a connection between the classification of a certain type of behaviour as a "mental illness" and the evaluation we make of the behaviour in question, and that the corresponding connection is lacking in the classification of problems as physical illnesses. Deviation from norms of biological function which (i.e. the deviation) is classified as illness could thus be in either direction, Szasz writes (for instance too many or too few white blood-cells), whereas similarly classified deviation from norms of behaviour is almost always in the "negative" direction — that is, in the direction of the immoral or the illegal. This implies, according to Szasz, that justifications are confused with explanations in ascriptions of "mental illness".

But Szasz is simply wrong here, as regards his premises as well as regards his conclusion, Brody states. Firstly one could argue that a person who washes his hands 200 times a day or a person who suffers from claustrophobia is acting neither immorally nor illegally, but is still regarded as mentally ill. Secondly it is not the case that every deviation from a biological norm is the same as physical illness. Brody puts forward unusual body heigth, unusually big nose and extremely red hair as examples. Thereby Szasz's premises would be refuted. But this is not all. Suppose that it were the case, Brody writes, that we only describe a behaviour as illness if we value it negatively. Does it follow from this that the concept of mental illness is merely a justification of our responses to the behaviour and does not also imply an explanation and/or description of it? No, because 'prescriptive' and 'descriptive' and/or 'explanatory' are not mutually exclusive concepts. A good apple, Brody suggests, has to satisfy descriptive criteria to be a good apple. But to call something a good apple also implies prescribing that you should choose it if you want a good apple. The same of course also applies to the concept of mental illness: it could well be prescriptive and descriptive. And thereby, Brody suggests, would also Szasz's conclusion have been proved false.

On this way of reasoning several comments must be made. Brody construes Szasz's premises as follows: 1) Only deviation from behavioural norms in the direction of immoral or illegal behaviour is viewed as "mental illness"; 2) All deviations from biological norms are physical illnesses. Thereafter he demonstrates that 1 as well as 2 is false. This construction of Szasz's premises seems arbitrary and wrongful. Szasz does not claim that all types of deviation from biological norms constitute illnesses. Nor does he claim that "mental illness" is always ascribed on the basis of deviations from behavioural norms in the direction of the immoral or the illegal. The starting point of his dicussion is that we speak of physical illnesses when we are dealing with deviations from biological norms, and that we speak of "mental illnesses" when we are dealing with deviations from certain behavioural norms. These basic assumptions Brody appears to accept. Furthermore Szasz, the way I read him, claims that an important difference can be noticed in ascriptions of physical illness and "mental illness", respectively, in that deviations from biological norms seemingly could happen in both directions and be called illnesses in either case, whereas ascriptions of "mental illness" in cases of deviation from behavioural norms are almost always made when the deviation is in one direction, more specifically the morally negatively valued one.

There is undoubtedly a problem in Szasz's account here, but a quite different one than Brody suggests. It could be questioned if ascriptions of "mental illness" are always made on the basis of behavioural deviations. Above (page 44) I made a distinction between two current uses of the term "mentally ill", that I shall here with some alteration repeat: 1) "mental illness" as a designation of conditions where the patient experiences suffering, functional disturbance or reduced capacity, and where the cause is assumed to be mental by nature, and 2) "mental illness" as a designation of behavioural deviations that, by someone other than the patient himself (his social surroundings, "society"), are perceived as disturbing, irrational, etc. (or as a designation of the supposed cause of those behaviours). With a very wide definition of "behavioural deviation" most (or all) instances of 1 could indeed be construed as instances of 2, but this would probably not be recommendable. Szasz's argument should reasonably be limited to apply to unambiguous instances of 2. You could rewrite and qualify the thesis he puts forward here, without changing too much its significance for the issue under discussion, as follows: When ascriptions of "mental illness" are made on the basis of deviations from behavioural norms, it seems not to be the case that if deviation in one direction from a certain norm is regarded as illness, deviation in the other direction is also regarded as illness. On closer examination we find that very often deviations in the direction of the immoral or the illegal are regarded as illnesses.

When Brody now presents a couple of examples of behavioural deviations that are not in the direction of the immoral or the illegal, this of course would have sufficed to refute the thesis that ascriptions of "mental illness" only are made when the deviation is in the direction of the immoral or the illegal (or the thesis that everything that is called "mental illness" is constituted by violations of moral norms). But this interpretation of Szasz's discussion is exceedingly narrow. What Brody ought to have presented, if he wanted to refute the main content of Szasz's argument, is a number of examples of illness-labelled behavioural deviations that really are in the direction of the immoral, and where deviations in the opposite direction are also regarded as illness!

With regard to Brody's attempt to demonstrate flawed logic in Szasz's transition to his conclusion, he successfully demonstrates that the concepts of prescriptive and descriptive and/or explanatory are not mutually exclusive, and that a concept (for instance the concept of mental illness) could well be prescriptive and descriptive and/or explanatory simultaneously. This is certainly most important, and it would of course be decisive to the discussion if Szasz had claimed that since the concept of mental illness is prescriptive it lacks descriptive or explanatory contents. But the claim that the prescriptive and descriptive functions of a concept are mutually exclusive is, as far as I have been able to find, not present in Szasz's reasoning, and the notion of such mutual exclusiveness is in no way necessary to pursue the argumentation that Szasz pursues on this issue. It is quite sufficient to suggest 1) that the prescriptive and the descriptive and/or explanatory functions of a concept can be kept distinguished in a meaningful way, 2) that the concept of mental illness serves primarily prescriptive functions, and 3) that the concept of mental illness is assumed to have descriptive and/or explanatory functions that it de facto lacks. Forceful objections to this should consist in demonstrating that the concept of mental illness serves primarily descriptive and/or explanatory functions and/or that the concept of mental illness does not function primarily as prescriptive/justificatory.

Brody concludes by saying that he does not know if Szasz is right or wrong, but that the argumentation Szasz provides is not able to prove his points. It seems not uncalled-for to suggest, on the contrary, that Szasz's criticism may well be open to valid objections, but that these could not be found among the ones supplied by Brody.

We have seen different critics object to Szasz's dichotomization of human problems into illnesses and "problems in living", and to his proposal that mental and behavioural disturbances should belong in the latter category, and this objection has been expressed partly by way of attempting to demonstrate prominent similarities between mental problems and physical illnesses, and partly by way of attempting to refute Szasz's suggestions of decisive differences. A third strategy is to claim that the two categories of problems (illnesses and "problems in living") are not mutually exclusive. This is suggested by Macklin,[25] Ausubel,[26] Ross[27] and Schoenfeld.[28] They seem to view this suggestion as an objection to the *logic* of Szasz's dichotomy. None of them, however, argues in much detail on this point. Ross speaks of "existential" problems developing so that they make the person ill. Ausubel suggests that when individuals for various reasons are unable to cope with "problems in living", they could react with severely disturbed or maladaptive behaviour. We should distinguish, however, between on the one hand a problem being simultaneously regarded as a "problem in living" and as an illness (which would be possible if the two categories were not mutually exclusive) and on the other hand a "problem in living" being the cause of illness (which is perfectly possible even if the two categories are mutually exclusive). Only the former concerns the logic of Szasz's dichotomy. That a pressing life-situation, troublesome social relations or exaggerated ambition, for instance, could cause a heart attack or an ulcer, would hardly be denied by Szasz, and would not imply that a meaningful drawing of the line between "problems in living" and illness could not be made.

The critics, however, really seem to be suggesting something quite different, viz. that the cognitive, emotional or behavioural problems that Szasz would place in the category of "problems in living", and thereby outside of the category of illnesses, really satisfy reasonable criteria of inclusion in the category of illnesses. The disagreement consists primarily in differing views on the proper definition of 'illness'. What they turn against, then, is not primarily the dichotomy of categories as such, but the criteria used to decide to which category a certain problem should belong. An alternative strategy would be to demarcate the category of "problems in living" in a different way. Schoenfeld,[29] for instance, seems to suggest that the class of "problems in living" includes the class of illnesses. But the purpose of Szasz's dichotomy is mainly to demonstrate that not all problems of social adjustment are medical by nature. In cases where difficulties of social adjustment are not caused by malfunctionings of the human body, we should, he suggests, not interpret the problems in medical terms, but rather in legal, political, ethical, social, etc. terms, and we should also not call those problems illnesses. The comprehensive term "problems in living" is perhaps less well-chosen, but this is hardly a logical problem.

Thereby we end this discussion of critical objections to the theses 2, 3 and 4. The discussion has perhaps provided certain opportunities to see more clearly the nature of the disagreements, rather than an unambiguous answer to the question of who is right. Szasz's theses may possibly appear somewhat less strong in some respects, in the light of criticism and alternative approaches, but they have not been substantially shaken. A reasonable conclusion from this part of the discussion is perhaps that the criticism directed against Szasz could probably be qualified in some respects, and that this is to be recommended to those who would claim to forcefully defend the concept of mental illness, but that no good reasons for Szasz to abandon his critical position have been found here.

Some concluding comments and reflections

The main purpose of the discussion in this chapter was to inquire into the extent to which Szasz's criticism of the concept of mental illness, and of the medical-model conception of abnormal behaviour and mental afflictions, could be defended against a number of current objections. Those objections were, mainly, discussed on the Szasz-opponent's own terms, and no attempts to qualify or improve the objections were made. It should not be denied that the amount of energy used to defend Szasz's criticism was greater than the amount used to find constructive elements in the attempts at objections provided by his opponents. A starting-point of this discussion was the intuition that Szasz's criticism contains valuable and important elements, and that a superficial waving aside of it would risk obscuring the fact that the conceptualization of mental afflictions and behavioural deviations in terms of "mental illness" is not self-evidently unproblematic. The discussion has shown, I believe, that several of the attempts made to refute Szasz's criticism are problematic, and that they cannot, in the form in which they have been presented, be taken to show that the critique is mistaken or groundless.

A short and summarizing overview of the discussion would now seem proper. On page 20 Szasz's criticism was formulated and specified in four theses, which were used — in (it is hoped) a clarifying way — as a basis of the discussion of objections. On pages 23-33 objections to Szasz's suggestion that the coming into being of the concept of mental illness is associated with a doubtful or mistaken enlargement of the concept of illness (thesis 1) were discussed. The disagreements among his critics as to in what way this thesis should be viewed as invalid, make the combined strength of the objections hard to assess. A problem in the assessment of this discussion is also that several writers in their reasonings seem to slide between on the one hand arguments based on analyses of contemporary medical and everyday usage, and on the other a wish to retroactively legitimize the changes that occurred during the 19th century concerning the concept of illness and concerning the classification of specific illnesses.

Several of the critics base their objections on the argument that the meaning of "illness" really always (or at least since antiquity) has been such that mental problems of diverse kinds in an unobjectionable way could be conceptualized in medical terms. Apart from the fact that this argument does not make any easier an explanation of the emergence of psychiatry as an established medical discipline, and the emergence of a demarcated class of "mental illnesses", during the 19th century, it could be argued to imply a neglecting of the importance of the growth of medical knowledge during the period preceding the emergence of psychiatry. The significance of "the scientific revolution" within medicine could be described as the illness being more clearly distinguished from the ill person, and medicine becoming focused more on treating the former than the latter. It seems reasonable to suppose that when psychiatry wanted to establish itself as a medical discipline, this "post-revolutionary" medical science constituted its model. Otherwise it becomes difficult to understand the intensive efforts to work out detailed nosological systems, the efforts to identify specific types and subtypes of "mental illnesses", and the experimenting to find specified treatment strategies for different "mental illnesses". The establishing of psychiatry as a medical discipline meant an abandoning of earlier, "pre-scientific" treatment efforts (like "moral treatment" along the lines of Tuke.). Psychiatry now was to become a medical science and practice, and the paradigm of its illness notions was primarily the view of disease or illness that now, around the middle of the 19th century, had made its break-through, and not the more abstract and diffuse illness notions of earlier centuries. To suggest, against this background, that the reclassification of behavioural and mental deviations can be viewed as something completely unproblematic, as certain of Szasz's opponents seem to do, appears less well-considered.

It does not seem unreasonable to suggest that there was some measure of liberty of choice, and that, without making some logical mistake, there was the possibility of choosing not to conceptualize in medical terms the phenomena subsequently classified as "mental illness". It should be noted in this context that neither the pointing out that there has taken place during the last 150 years a transferral of a number of human problems and behavioural deviations to the class of (mental) illnesses, nor the notion that this reclassification demanded some sort of change in the meaning of "illness", is in any way unique to Szasz. This description of the state of affairs is often the starting-point of various contributions to the debate on psychiatry, and the disagreements largely consist in differences of opinion as to whether those changes should be viewed as scientifically legitimate and socially to be wished for or not. Szasz's view, as we have seen, is that no sound scientific or logical reasons for the change has been supplied, and that the motives probably were not of a scientific character. That his critics should have succeeded in proving him wrong on this point I find it hard to see.

On pages 33-53 a number of arguments against theses 2, 3 and 4 were discussed. We have seen how Szasz's dichotomization of human problems into illnesses and "problems in living" (thesis 4) has been the object of questionings that aim at demonstrating that no distinct demarcation line could be drawn between those categories. Particularly the demarcation criterion that is based on Szasz's proposition that the meaning of "illness" is, or ought to be, physico-chemical disturbance of the human body (thesis 2) has been objected to, but also Szasz's suggestions of important differences in ascriptions of physical and "mental" illness, respectively, (thesis 3) have been questioned.

A central element of the argumentation of several critics is the proposition that "illness" or "disease" primarily refers to suffering, incapacitation, reduced functioning or the like, but that no association with physical disturbance need be assumed. We have, however, not encountered any ambitious attempt at arguing for this proposition, or at demonstrating the resonableness of it. The argumentation therefore becomes problematic in several ways. On the one hand this suggestion of characterizing the meaning of "illness" is not able to demarcate the class of illnesses in a reasonable way, and on the other it seems to exclude some of the mental problems that one would want to include in the class of illnesses. The conclusion from this part of the discussion must therefore be that forceful objections to Szasz require a substantially more developed and qualified argumentation in favour of the proposition that the concept of illness does not contain, and should not contain, any reference to physical abnormality, as well as in favour of the proposition that it should be defined in terms of suffering or incapacitation.

We have also seen some attempts at showing through comparisons and analogies that different emotional problems and behavioural disturbances are similar to physical illnesses to the extent that they could well be classified as illnesses. Problematic aspects of this way of reasoning are on the one hand that one, without telling why, directly chooses to observe similarities rather than differences, and on the other that one gets into trouble when it comes to showing that the aspects of comparison chosen are really relevant to decisions concerning whether or not a certain phenomenon is a disease phenomenon. A substantial confusion is also created in this context by the obscurity on the part of several writers as to what the term "mental illness" should really be taken to refer to. On the one hand it is suggested that the term primarily describes a behaviour as such rather than a cause of it. This position seems determined primarily by the wish to escape a discussion of "mental illness" in terms of a mental "disease entity" inherent within the individual. But on the other hand there seems to be an unwillingness to see that this use of the term obviously comes into conflict with everyday as well as medical usage. To sum up, I believe we must conclude that the objections to theses 2, 3 and 4 here presented would not supply any compelling refutation of Szasz's criticism. But does this imply that his criticism is correct and unobjectionable? On this we cannot be certain. The discussion has left us with a number of implicit and hinted-at notions in the arguments of the opponents of Szasz, of a modernized and developed medical model that would allow for the unobjectionable conceptualization of mental afflictions and behavioural disturbances in terms of mental illness. The articulation and qualification of that model, and of the notions of illness that it is built on, would seem to be an important task with regard to the achievement of a more thorough assessment of the real strength of the Szaszian type of criticism of the concept of mental illness.

Notes

1 Schoenfeld, C. G.: An Analysis of the Views of Thomas Szasz, in Vatz, R. E. and Weinberg, L. S. (eds.): *Thomas Szasz: Primary Values and Major Contentions*, New York, 1983.

2 Macklin, R: Mental Health and Mental Illness: Some Problems of Definition and Concept formation.

3 Margolis, J.: The Concept of Mental Illness: A Philosophical Examination.

4 Pies, R.: On Myths and Countermyths, in Vatz, R. E. and Weinberg, L. S. (eds.): *Thomas Szasz: Primary Values and Major Contentions*.

5 Roth, M.: Schizophrenia and the Theories of Thomas Szasz, in *British Journal of Psychiatry*, 129, 1976, pp. 317-326.

6 Ross, A.: Opgør med antipsykiatrien, in *Bibliotek for Laeger*, 171, 4, 1979, pp. 241-267.

7 Szasz's account of the history of the coming into being of the notion of mental illness is controversial and somewhat difficult to interpret. He sometimes writes in

a way that seems to suggest that the very term "mental illness" was created in the 19th century. But this would certainly be an incorrect suggestion. The term "mental illness", or its equivalent, can probably be traced far back in antiquity. The core of his argument, however, rests on the contention that changes took place in the 19th century that brought into being psychiatry as a specific medical subdiscipline, distinguished from neurology, and with a specific class of "mental diseases", distinguished from physical diseases, as its legitimate area of expertise. These changes, according to Szasz, had a major impact on the issue of what kind of phenomena can be conceptualized in medical terms and brought under medical jurisdiction. He certainly shares this contention with other contributors to the discussion of psychiatry. (See, for instance, Conrad, P and Schneider, J. W: *The Medicalization of Deviance*.)

8 Ausubel, D. P.: Personality Disorder Is Disease, in Scheff, T. (ed.): *Mental Illnesses and Social Processes*.

9 Pies, R.: On Myths and Countermyths, in Vatz, R. E. and Weinberg, L. S. (eds.): *Thomas Szasz: Primary Values and Major Contentions*.

10 Roth, M.: Schizophrenia and the Theories of Thomas Szasz.

11 Ibid.

12 Pies, R.: On Myths and Countermyths.

13 Macklin, R.: Mental Health and Mental Illness: Some Problems of Definition and Concept Formation.

14 Margolis, J.: The Concept of Mental Illness: A Philosophical Examination.

15 Ausubel, D.: Personality Disorder Is Disease.

16 Margolis, J.: The Concept of Mental Illness: A Philosophical Examination, p. 7.

17 Moore, M. S.: Some Myths about "Mental Illness", in Vatz, R. E. and Weinberg, L. S. (eds.): *Thomas Szasz: Primary Values and Major Contentions*.

18 Macklin, R: Mental Health and Mental Illness: Some Problems of Definition and Concept Formation.

19 Redlich, F. C. and Freedman, D. X.: *The Theory and Practice of Psychiatry*.

20 Moore, M. S.: Some Myths about "Mental Illness".

21 Ibid. p. 191.

22 Ibid. p. 190.

23 Brody, B.: Szasz on Mental Illness, in Caplan, A. L., Engelhardt, H. T., Jr. and McCartney, J. J. (eds.).: *Concepts of Health and Disease*.

24 Ibid. p. 475.

25 Macklin, R.: Mental Health and Mental Illness: Some Problems of Definition and Concept Formation.

26 Ausubel, D. P.: Personality Disorder Is Disease.

27 Ross, A.: Opgør med antipsykiatrien.

28 Schoenfeld, C. G.: An Analysis of the Views of Thomas Szasz.

29 Ibid.

4 On medical models

Introduction

The discussion of a number of recurrent objections to the Szaszian type of critique has left us with no clear picture of the status of the medical-model conception of abnormal behaviour and mental afflictions. And it has certainly not provided any firm ground for refuting the critique. If we were to leave the discussion at this point, it would be with a feeling that the Szaszian position might well be quite reasonable. The strategy now, however, will be to pursue the analysis some steps further. I shall do this by way of abandoning the strategy of discussion adopted in chapter 3; the one, that is, of discussing the arguments of the opponents of Szasz on their own terms, just as they stand. I shall try to articulate and qualify some of their arguments to get a somewhat more substantial sense of the possibilities of forcefully counterarguing the critique of the medical-model conception of abnormal behaviour and mental afflictions. Some very loosely articulated implications and hints in the reasonings of the opponents of Szasz will be taken seriously in an effort to see if these implications and hints could be qualified and elaborated upon. The overall strategy of trying to problematize the medical-model conception will, however, in no way be abandoned.

In chapter 5 I shall try to critically assess two elaborated medical models with regard to their application to abnormal behaviour and mental afflictions. The key question will be whether a concept of *mental disease* could be reasonably constructed on the platform of either one of those models. The two models will be introduced in ideal-type form and elaborated upon in this chapter. I shall begin the chapter, however, with some remarks on the recurrent claim that Szasz and other critics build their objections to the medical-model conception of so-called mental-illness phenomena on a false representation of the medical model. I shall also, as a prerequisite to the introduction of the two models and to the main discussions in the next chapter, make some necessary distinctions and clarifications, primarily pertaining to the notions of model and medical model.

On the existence of an established medical model and on the quest for a revised one

One often recurring objection to Szasz and other critics of the application of a medical model to mental and behavioural problems is that they base their critique on an oversimplified or even false account of the nature of the medical model that is operative in discourse on health and disease in general. It is sometimes argued that it is through making a caricature of "the medical model" and the accepted notions of "ordinary" disease or illness and health that Szasz and others can build a case for rejecting the extension of medical-model reasoning to include behavioural and mental abnormalities. Particularly the Szaszian notion that "disease", within "ordinary" medical-model reasoning, must refer to some organic, problem-generating, abnormality is questioned and rejected. This kind of questioning of Szasz's premises could be interpreted along somewhat different lines. It could be taken to imply that Szasz's construal of the medical model is flawed in *some* crucial respects, for instance when it comes to specifying the precise characteristics of disease or illness. This would then be compatible with the view that there is something that could be referred to as *the* medical model, but that this something is far more complex and intricate than the Szaszian account implies. But the objections could also take the form of proposing that there is not *one* medical model, but that there are at least two, and that Szasz's critique, by taking it that the notion of a medical model is singular and consensual, oversimplifies the discussion. And a third interpretation of the scepticism towards Szasz's notion of a medical model could be made along the lines that the medical model that Szasz depicts is out-of-date and on its way to becoming non-existent and being completely replaced by a "modern" one, with very different basic concepts of health and illness as corner-stones.

One sometimes gets the feeling, when reading critical reviews of Szasz's writings along these lines, that Szasz and a handful of other critics are the only upholders of an out-dated, or non-existent, or fundamentally misinterpreted version of "the medical model". But this, I would claim, is not correct. The notion of a medical model, where organic abnormality is a strongly stressed necessary condition of disease and where medicine is viewed as the art and science of dealing with "body-machine-faults", is actually prevalent among writers with very diverging views on the medical-model conception of so-called mental illnesses. Among critics of that conception it is dominant, of course, and a list of critical writers upholding this view would be fatiguingly long. But equally among apologists of psychiatry as a medical discipline, and of mental and behavioural abnormalities as "mental illnesses", this view is current.

I shall give some examples that substantiate what I have just said, and that also point to two diverging ways of reacting, among defenders of the medical-model conception of so-called mental-illness phenomena, to the critique. Ludwig,[1] on the question of how psychiatry should react to the critical views of the concept of mental illness, argues forcefully for the need of psychiatry, if it is to maintain its credibility as a medical discipline, to step firmly back into a traditional biological-medical framework, where, according to him, the only reasonable basis for construing "mental illness" as a medical problem lies. Strongly opposing current tendencies to enlarge the domain of psychiatric expertise to encompass diverse kinds of character disorders, social maladjustment reactions, dependency syndromes, existential depressions etc., Ludwig suggests that psychiatric disease or mental illness should be defined as "any debilitating, cognitive-affective-behaviour disorder due primarily to known, suggestive or presumed biological brain dysfunctions, either biochemical or neurophysiological in nature."[2] So, according to Ludwig, psychiatry should react to the critique by tightening its bonds to "ordinary" medical thinking. It should limit its responsibilities, and its legitimate domain of expertise, to the medical model which, writes Ludwig, is distinguished from non-medical models by dealing with symptoms and signs of patients — symptoms and signs, that is, of disease, which in turn is due to known or unknown natural, rather than metapsychological, interpersonal or social causes. Obviously Ludwig founds his suggestions concerning the future course of psychiatry on a notion of the nature of *the* medical model that is quite similar to the one suggested by Szasz.

Engel[3] exemplifies an almost contradictory reaction to the "anti-psychiatric" critique. To hold on to psychiatry's threatened status as a medical discipline, he suggests that not psychiatry but the medical model should be changed. The prevalent bio-medical view of disease should be abandoned in favour of a new medical model, with a new conception of disease, that would benefit psychiatry (which could then remain an unproblematic medical discipline) as well as medicine in general (which would acquire an updated conception of disease, that, according to Engel, is badly needed). I shall have more to say about Engel's suggestions presently, but for now it suffices to note that Engel too presupposes and acknowledges the existence of the medical model that Szasz uses to point out the unreasonableness of viewing "mental illness" as a disease-type problem.

This should suffice to refute the notion that Szasz's version of the medical model is an imaginary and misconceived construction. I believe it is safe to propose that many medical men, biologically oriented psychiatrists as well as physicians in general, would define disease roughly the way Szasz does. And I think it is not out of the way to regard various suggestions with regard to changing the medical model (where Engel's proposal is but one example) as implicit acknowledgements of the existence of a model along the Szaszian lines of description. So it would be, at least, incorrect to suggest that Szasz and other critics rest their case on a *caricatural* construction of the medical model. Quite a different thing is that there seems to be opposition to this prevalent medical model. There are suggestions of reforming, reformulating or even abandoning it. And one important reason to replace or revise the biologically based, "machine-fault", medical model is undoubtedly that this would make the application of medical discourse to "mental-illness-type" phenomena less controversial. How could a modernized medical model be constructed, that would allow for unobjectionable inclusion of the "mental-illness" type of abnormal behaviour and mental afflictions? There are several suggestions flourishing in the debate. An often recurring theme is the proclaimed need of taking into account dimensions other than hard-fact biological malfunctioning when defining disease or illness. The suffering- and incapacitation-dimensions of disease-problems should be stressed to a far greater extent than is the case in the prevalent medical-model reasoning, it is suggested. I shall, in this context, bypass the sometimes expressed notion that *all* kinds of human suffering and incapacitation, by their very nature as suffering and incapacitation, are suitable for inclusion in the medical model, which I believe to be hopelessly counter-intuitive, and eventually discuss two elaborated suggestions of how a medical model capable of including so-called mental-illness phenomena could be constructed. First, however, a certain way of misconstruing the issue of the need of a new or revised medical model should be commented upon.

There is a particular way of confusing the motive of wishing to make medical-model reasoning applicable to the "mental illness" type of phenomena with motives of quite a different nature. Engel[4] exemplifies this. He takes his point of departure in the discussion within psychiatry of "the crisis of psychiatry", and of various suggestions of how to solve it. The crisis he speaks of is one of uncertainty and ambiguity as to psychiatry's status as a medical discipline and to the status of the "mental illness" type of phenomena as diseases. The problem as many psychiatrists see it is, according to Engel, that psychiatry has tended to be concerned with a heterogeneous grouping of psychosocial problems and issues which seem to lie outside of medicine's responsibility and authority. Engel distinguishes two ways out of this dilemma that have been proposed in the debate. Either psychiatry could take seriously the Szaszian type of critique and step out of medicine to become a behavioural, non-medical discipline. Or it could, along the lines suggested by Ludwig, reviewed above, tighten its bonds with medicine proper by eschewing responsibility for every kind of psychosocial problem that is not believed, or proven, to be due to biological dysfunction. Engel then goes on to reject both ways, and suggests, as mentioned above, that it is the medical model, not psychiatry, that is in need of change. The dominant model of disease today, he writes, is biomedical and assumes disease to be fully accounted for by deviation from biological variables. But this model, he suggests, has outlived its value, and should be replaced by a "bio-psycho-social" model, taking into account psychological and social variables and dimensions of illness. And as far as I can see, Engel contends that this would provide arguments against the position that "mental illness is a myth" on account of its non-conformance to the concept of disease in general. But the arguments he supplies in favour of this contention actually achieve nothing of the kind.

Engel makes a comparison between what he takes to be two well-established diseases — one physical, diabetes, and one mental, schizophrenia — to show that they are completely analogous along a number of dimensions. In both cases the presence of a biochemical defect "at best defines a necessary but not a sufficient condition for the occurrence of the human experience of the disease, the illness."[5] Furthermore, he writes, the variability in the clinical expressions of diabetes and schizophrenia requires that psychological, social and cultural factors be taken into account in order for each of them to be fully understood. The two diseases are equally analogous in that behavioural and psychosocial knowledge is required to establish relationships between the biochemical processes and the clinical data. Diabetes and schizophrenia are also analogous in that psychological and social factors influence the onset and the course of both. And, he notes, psychological and social factors are, in both diseases, crucial in determining whether and when patients will come to view themselves, or be viewed by others, as sick. In both cases "rational treatment" that is only directed at the biochemical abnormality will not suffice to restore the patient to health. For this, psychological and social factors are also required. And, finally, in both cases the psychological and social dimensions of the physician's behaviour and of the physician-patient relationship are of great importance to therapeutic success.

So, Engel argues, in cases of physical as well as in cases of mental disease, psychosocial factors are extremely important to provide "a basis for understanding the determinants of disease and aiming at rational treatments and patterns of health-care".[6] Therefore we need a biopsychosocial model of disease to replace the "dogmatic" biomedical model.

And all this looks perfectly reasonable, of course. But it provides not a shred of argument against the Szaszian position. Engel starts out with what looks like the intention of showing that the problems called "mental illnesses" could be shown to be disease-type problems, if we change, or "modernize", the medical model in a certain direction, and ends up with a defence of the importance of taking into account psychological and social aspects of disease-problems. He seems to confuse two issues: 1) the question of what should be viewed as disease and what should not — that is, what problems, or parts of problems should be viewed as belonging to the category of diseases — and 2) the question of what people who are diseased (and undoubtedly a lot of other people also) need in terms of care, understanding, psychological and social support, etc.

The point is that the only disease-distinguishing factor in the list of analogous factors in diabetes and schizophrenia supplied by Engel is the biochemical abnormality. Or, at least, there is nothing in his account that would suggest the existence of any other such factor. If Engel wanted to show that mental or behavioural abnormalities that are excluded from disease-status with the biomedical model could reasonably be included in the category of diseases with his proposed biopsychosocial model, he would have to show that psychological and social factors are in themselves sufficient to establish the disease-status of human problems. As far as I can see, there is nothing that stands in the way of agreeing that doctors should consider social and psychological factors in the context of illness-problems (and be trained to do so), that doctors should bear in mind that the patient is a person and not just a body, that the problems of illness have important psychological and social dimensions, *and* at the same time to hold the view that disease should be defined in terms of structural or functional disorder of the human organism.

So the kind of modernized or revised medical model hinted at by opponents to Szasz in chapter 3 would have to be constructed along lines very different from Engel's biopsychosocial model. We shall presently approach closer the features of such a model. But first some elaborations on the notion of model are required.

On models, fundamentalism and metaphorism: Some distinctions and clarifications

Before approaching some suggestions of how "the medical model" could be more stringently formulated and articulated, some important distinctions and clarifications should be made as prerequisites of the discussions to follow. First, taking the cue from Szasz's claim that "mental illness" is a metaphor, I shall distinguish between two radically different ways of arguing for the appropriateness of using the term "mental illness": a *fundamentalist* and a *metaphorist* way. The fundamentalist argument claims that so-called mental illnesses are illnesses in exactly the same sense that "ordinary", or physical, illnesses are illnesses. This involves espousing the notion that there is a general concept of illness, such that the central, defining, characteristics of that concept are shared by the sub-concepts of physical illness and mental illness. The metaphorist argument rests on the notion that "mental illnesses" are not illnesses in a genuine sense. This involves acknowledging that so-called mental-illness problems lack some (or all) of the defining characteristics of the general concept of illness and that they therefore differ, on crucial points, from the phenomena called "ordinary", or physical illnesses. But, according to the metaphorist argument, there are some good reasons for viewing "mental-illness" problems *as if* they really were illnesses. Those reasons would then, typically, turn out to be of an extra-theoretical nature.

This distinction somewhat reflects the two lines of argumentation, for and against the appropriateness of the concept of mental illness, presented in chapter 1: a "philosophical" and an "ideological" one. The major parts of the discussions to follow in chapter 5 will be focused on the reasonableness or otherwise of the fundamentalist approach. In the final chapter of the study I shall have some things to say about the metaphorist approach.

The most frequently used expression in the polemics over the dilemma of "mental illness" is probably "the medical model". It is this model, or rather the use of it in the context of "mental illness" problems, that is the target of the critique, and it is this model that the protagonists of the mental-illness concept defend. But the model discussion is to some extent confused by an ambiguity as to the meaning of "model", which I believe could be avoided by making a simple distinction. I shall distinguish between two kinds of models: *conceptual* models and *explanatory* models. A conceptual model is a system of interrelated concepts used to characterize, and categorize, and direct us to view in a certain way, the nature or essence of certain phenomena. An explanatory model is used to explain phenomena, for instance by attributing causes to them. A conceptual model could (theoretically) be compatible with any number of explanatory models, each providing a separate kind of explanation. To use a conceptual model need not imply any bias whatsoever as regards the explanation of the phenomena to which the model is applied. In most cases, however, a conceptual model will only be compatible with a limited number of explanatory models, because certain references to cause-attribution are built into the central concepts of the model.

I believe this distinction can help us avoid some confusion. The expression "medical model" can then, according to the distinction, be used in two different senses. In the "mental illness" debate it is quite often used in a narrow explanatory sense. "The medical model" then refers to a certain way of explaining so-called mental-illness problems in terms of physico-chemical disturbances. This usage often goes hand in hand with a misrepresentation, or too limited a notion, of what it could mean to be opposed to the medical model of "mental illness" problems. If "medical model" is used in a conceptual-model sense it refers to a characterization of certain phenomena in terms of illness or disease. This conceptual model could subsume diverse notions of how the phenomena should be explained (in terms of physico-chemical variables, in terms of psychological variables, in terms of psychosocial variables, etc.). So you could be opposed to "the medical model" either in an explanatory-model sense, for instance because you regard the attempts to explain "mental illnesses" the same way that "ordinary" illnesses are typically explained as unsuccessful or unlikely to succeed, or you could be opposed to "the medical model" in a conceptual-model sense, for instance because you regard it as inappropriate to conceptualize so-called mental-illness phenomena in terms of illness or disease. The distinction also leaves room for the possibility that you could be opposed to the explanation of "mental illness" phenomena in terms of biomedical variables while still accepting the application of a conceptual medical model to those phenomena, provided that you espouse a definition of the concept of disease or illness in terms other than biomedical.

Analogously a lot of confusion, regarding the expressions "social model", "sociological model", and variants of those, could be avoided by keeping the distinction clear between the two kinds of models. You could talk of sociological models of "mental illness" problems in the sense of explanatory models containing specific assumptions concerning the causes of "mental illnesses", often also including assumptions regarding their symptomatology and correct treatment. The application of such a model could be quite compatible with the notion that "mental illnesses" are illness-type problems, even though it would imply a disagreement as to their being appropriately explained in, for instance, biological or bio-chemical terms. To apply a sociological *conceptual* model would, however, mean something completely different. "Mental illness" problems would then be conceptualized, not in medical, but in sociological terms, and the application of such a model would entail regarding the problems in question as something other than illnesses.

Two ideal-type medical models

The above distinctions have, it is hoped, made us better prepared to discuss some elaborated medical models of abnormal behaviour and mental afflictions. When it comes to models of "mental illness", or madness, or deviant behaviours, the literature abounds with suggestions as to how such models should be characterized, typified or distinguished. Since a failure to keep the conceptual-explanatory distinction clear is very frequent in those suggestions, and since they on that account tend to be rather unfruitful and unsatisfactory from the point of view of the purposes of this study, I shall bypass them all and go on to make my own model-characterizations in a way that will suit the approach of this analysis.

Taking seriously the implications and suggestions inherent in the objections to Szasz's critique that were discussed in chapter 3, I shall propose a distinction between two conceptual medical models that differ substantially along certain crucial dimensions. Each of them will then be assessed with regard to its possibilities of supplying grounds for a fundamentalist conception of abnormal behaviour and mental afflictions in terms of "mental disease" that (i. e. the conception) would not run into the kind of difficulties we found with the arguments supplied by Szasz's opponents in the previous chapter. I shall, for lack of better terms, name them "the traditional medical model" (the TMM) and "the modern(ized) medical model" (the MMM). An ideal-typical characterization of the differences between them will run as follows. The TMM is focused on causes, or on "the cause-side" of the health-disease complex. To say that a phenomenon is a disease-type phenomenon is here necessarily to say that a certain kind of cause of human problems is present. And it is quite possible to say that a very similar problem is not a disease-type phenomenon, when the cause of the problem is of another type. The MMM, on the other hand, is focused on effects or consequences, or on the "effect-side" of the health-disease complex. To say that a phenomenon is a disease-type phenomenon is here necessarily to say that a certain type of effect or consequence is present. And it is quite possible to say that a similar phenomenon is not a disease-type phenomenon if its consequences are different. The TMM is reductionist in the sense that the characterization of a phenomenon as a disease-type phenomenon is accomplished by way of expressing the nature of higher-level (more complex) circumstances in terms of lower-level (more basic) circumstances. The MMM, on the other hand, is holistic in the sense that the characterization of a phenomenon as a disease-type phenomenon is accomplished by way of expressing the nature of lower-level (more basic) circumstances in terms of higher-level (more complex) circumstances. The TMM framework is built on the notion that the disease-concept is value-free, while the MMM framework includes the notion that the disease-concept is value-loaded. And, finally, within TMM-reasoning health and disease are contradictory and mutually exclusive notions, while this is not the case within MMM-reasoning.

This, it seems to me, should cover the essential dimensions on which disagreement over the nature of a medical model (a conceptual medical model, that is) would be possible. The objections to the Szaszian type of criticism of the medical-model conception of abnormal behaviour and mental afflictions could then be articulated either on the grounds that he correctly presupposes a TMM-oriented medical model to be the one prevalent in general medical discourse, but that he misconstrues the more precise specification of its key concepts, or on the grounds that he fails to realize that the correct way of characterizing health and disease is along MMM-oriented lines.

To somewhat substantiate the rather abstract, and ideal-typical, outline of the two differing kinds of medical models, and to provide us with a set of more specific schemata for characterizing health and disease in general, I shall give a few examples of medical-philosophical theorizing. These will then in chapter 5 serve as platforms for a renewed testing out of the criticism of the medical-model conception of abnormal behaviour and mental afflictions.

Two TMM-inclined theories of health and disease

The best articulated example of a TMM-inclined theory of health and disease, to my knowledge, is the one put forward by Christopher Boorse.[7] A quite similar view is presented by Alf Ross.[8] The theories of health and disease put forward by these philosophers come close to what might be described as sophisticated versions of what in the debate has sometimes been called "the faulty-machine model" of disease.

Let us start with Boorse's theory. The core concepts around which he builds his theory are 'biological function' and 'statistical normality'. Strongly opposing current notions of disease decisions as inescapably value-laden, Boorse proposes that disease is a value-neutral concept. To state that something should be included in the class of diseases is to state a matter of scientific judgement of facts, not to express a value-judgement of this something. Health is normality, and the normal is the natural. Disease (which is the opposite of health) is that which interferes with the natural, and such interference it is possible to detect empirically and state objectively. To work his way to this view, which he claims to be in strong accord with ordinary and medical usage, Boorse argues as follows. Species of living organisms are products of evolution. The result of this evolution is, for every species, a natural design, a species-typical design, which comprises the hierarchy of interlocking functional systems that supports the life of organisms of that type. Those biological designs have a strong consistency over time, and it is precisely on this consistency that medical theory and practice rely. So a species-design is, in other words, a uniformity of biological functional organization, typical of members of the species in question.

Now, a function in this context is a contribution to a goal. Organisms are goal-directed; they change their behaviours to adapt to circumstantial changes, so as to maintain their contributions to the attainment of certain results. "In fact", Boorse writes, "the structure of organisms shows a mean-end hierarchy with goal-directedness at every level."[9] And the function of any part or process of an organism is its ultimate contribution to certain superordinate goals of the organism as a whole. In the health/disease discussion, Boorse suggests, the ultimate goals towards the attainment of which biological functions contribute are survival and reproduction. The next step, then, is to answer the question: How do we discover a species design and how do we establish what are the typical characteristics of it? And this is where the notion of statistical normality comes into the picture. That which is typical of a certain function of some part of the organism is typical in a statistical sense. It is through empirically establishing the statistically normal functioning (that is, the contributing to survival and reproduction) of an organ that we can arrive at statements about the species design. We should further note that normal functionings, in this sense, show some natural variations within a species owing to sex and age. The statistical abstractions on which normal functioning is established should therefore be made, not from the total population of a species, but from age groups of a sex within a species.

Within this framework Boorse is then able to define the concepts of disease and health more precisely. Health is the same as normal functional ability, which is to say the ability of each internal part of a member of the species to function normally — that is, to contribute to survival and reproduction with at least typical efficiency. Disease is a type of internal state which impairs health, in the sense that it reduces one or more functional abilities below the efficiency that is typical of an age group of a sex within a species.

As already mentioned, 'disease' in this theory is a theoretical, value-neutral, concept. Decisions regarding health and disease are objectively grounded matters of stating of facts. The same, however, is not true of ascriptions of illness to a person. Boorse distinguishes between disease and illness. The distinction could be described as one between opposites of two distinguishable notions of health. In one sense health is a theoretical concept. This is the notion of normal biological functioning described above. The opposite of this sense of "health" is disease. But in another sense health is a "practical" concept. Medicine is not just a theoretical discipline, but also (and from some points of view even primarily) a practical one. And within the context of practical suffering-ameliorating medicine health is certainly something desirable. The opposite of health within this medical-practical framework is therefore something undesirable. And this something undesirable is what is, according to Boorse, called illness. Now, through the use of this distinction we could retain the notion of disease as something value-free, something that can be expressed in neutral, objective terms, and yet at the same time retain the notion that to be ill, to have an illness, is something bad. The relations between the notions of disease and illness are then explained by Boorse as follows. "A disease is an *illness* only if it is serious enough to be incapacitating and therefore is 1) undesirable for its bearer; 2) a title to special treatment, and 3) a valid excuse for normally criticizable behaviour."[10] This means that the class of disease-phenomena is larger than, and contains, the class of illness-phenomena. There could be, and there are, disease-instances that are not at the same time illness-instances. A person can be diseased without being ill. But, and this is important, disease is a necessary condition of illness. We can only speak of illness when there is disease present.

Now we turn to Ross's approach. Disease, Ross suggests, seems to have something to do with a breakdown of a certain presupposed "order of nature". The difficult question to answer is what kind of "order" is here implied. To approach an explication of our intuitions of this order, Ross presents an analogy. Let us suppose, he writes, that people with substantial knowledge of physics and mechanics were to come into contact with a thing that they had never seen before, namely a car. By studying this object they would be able to gradually achieve an understanding of the various parts of it and to realize that there were functions to be supplied by these, and furthermore that these functions could work together towards a certain purpose: the driving of the car. And if the car stopped working they would equally be able to investigate the nature of the problem that caused the malfunctioning. They would be able to grasp the plan of organization or functioning of the car.

Now, Ross proposes, in the same way a plan of functioning could be arrived at with reference to the human organism; a plan of normality of functioning of the human body. There is however some difference between the way we arrive at the plan of human normal functioning and the way the plan of the car was arrived at. We could not grasp the plan of normality of the human body by way of studying one individual. The plan of normality is a plan of the biological structure and functions of the human species. It is by studying the functioning of a certain part of the human organism in a great number of individuals that we can arrive at the understanding of the plan of functioning of the species of humans. But what will certainly not be found is the existence in each and every part of the individual human organism of a complete working according to the plan of biological functioning of the species. This is why the plan is in one sense an ideal-plan. The plan expresses the normal functioning of an ideal human organism, where each part of the organism conforms to the plan.

On the basis of this Ross is now in a position to tentatively define the notion of disease. To state that a person is somatically diseased, Ross writes, means to state that he is in a state where his bodily functions do not run in accordance with the plan of normality of the species, with regard taken to sex and age. If a person is diseased he will in most cases experience the disease in certain ways. He will experience suffering and incapacitation, which should then be viewed as signs and symptoms of the disease's presence. But, Ross notes, there are also instances of latent disease — that is, disease without accompanying symptoms and signs. And, finally, to say that a person suffers from a specific somatic disease means to say that he is diseased in the sense defined above and that the characteristics of the disease could be subsumed under one of the disease-entities of clinical medicine.

Obviously the two theories of health and disease just reviewed are strongly resemblant of each other. There are some differences of expression, and also some differences of substance, but those are of little consequence to our subsequent discussion. Let us, before we turn our attention to some opposing, MMM-inclined, theories, have a summary of the main features of the theories of Ross and Boorse, and an inclination of some aspects of them to bear in mind till the next chapter. An important feature of the theories is the heavy reliance on the notion of normal functioning. And the normality of the normal functioning is tied to the notion of empirical investigation of the workings of the human organism. Disease-judgements are, with these theories, not evaluative. It is possible to state, in scientific, objective and neutral terms, that a phenomenon is a disease-type phenomenon, or that a person is diseased. In some cases of disease (or, perhaps more accurately, in the majority of them) the presence of disease in a person is accompanied by distress, suffering and incapacitation. This part of the complex of having a disease, which Boorse distinguishes as the illness-requirements and Ross speaks of as the experience-aspect of disease, is surely a matter of (dis-)value.

Three MMM-inclined theories of health and disease

Now let us turn our attention to a set of theories of health and disease that operate on quite different grounds and that exemplify and substantiate what I have termed MMM-inclined reasoning about the health-illness complex. These theories stress that human beings are individuals acting in a context of social relations. The key features of health and disease, on this view, are that they affect a person as a whole. The restrictions a disease puts on a person's range of possibilities of action are not only stressed, but actually, in ways that will presently be referred to, made the *defining* characteristics of disease.

Ingmar Pörn[11] has proposed a theory of health which he terms "the equilibrium theory". The key notion of the theory is that of a requirement of a balance, or equilibrium, between on the one hand a person's resources for action, his abilities, and on the other hand the goals the person wants to reach. We should speak of health when a person's repertoire, the sum total of his abilities, exactly matches his profile of goals. It is important to notice that the repertoire of a person should be kept distinct from the opportunities of action that are at hand. A person may not be able to act in a way that his intrapersonal resources would allow, because opportunities of action are lacking or inadequate. This, of course, would not make us question his health. Illness, which is the opposite of health in this theory, is defined as the state of a person which obtains when his repertoire (by which is meant his intrapersonal resources) is inadequate relative to his profile of goals.This makes health and illness matters of the person as a whole. Disease is not, within this scheme of reasoning, the opposite of health (just as health is not the same as the absence of disease). Diseases are defined as processes that have a causal tendency to restrict repertoires and thereby to compromise health. But, as I understand this theory, there could surely be disease-instances that do not affect the health of a person, precisely because they do not make inadequate his repertoire relative to his profile of goals.

A similar theory has been put forward by Caroline Whitbeck.[12] Health is characterized by her as "the psychophysiological capacity to act or respond appropriately in a wide variety of situations."[13] And "appropriately" here means "in a way that is supportive of, or at least minimally destructive to, the agent's goals, projects, aspirations and so forth."[14] This, obviously, is in accord with Pörn's reasoning. Whitbeck strongly stresses that disease and health are concepts of different orders. Health is something over and above the absence of disease. This also means that a high degree of health is compatible with having a disease. Disease, in Whitbeck's scheme, is somewhat lengthily defined as follows. Diseases are 1) psychophysiological processes that 2) compromise people's ability to do what they commonly want and expect to be able to do, and that 3) are not necessary in order for people to do what they commonly want to be able to do, and that 4) are either statistically abnormal in those at risk or there is some other ground for a reasonable hope of finding ways to treat or prevent them in an effective way. This entails viewing disease as something relative to a societal context. The ability that diseases are said to compromise is people's ability to do what people commonly want to do, which of course is a matter of variation among different social settings. The notion of disease is value-laden in Whitbeck's theory, but in a sense that differs somewhat from the sense in which 'health' is value-laden. While 'health' is value-laden in a strong sense, 'disease', Whitbeck suggests, is value-laden in a "capability-sense". This means that disease belongs to a category of phenomena that people ordinarily want to be able to control and avoid. This, however, does not exclude the possibility that an individual might, for some personal reasons, value positively some instance of disease.

Finally, let us review a third MMM-inclined theory of health, proposed by Lennart Nordenfelt.[15] Nordenfelt, in accord with Pörn and Whitbeck, takes the notion of health to be the primary, or more basic, notion in the health-disease complex and eventually arrives at a definition of disease in terms of health-compromising factors. Health is defined as a person's ability to reach his vital goals. Nordenfelt recognizes that two kinds of phenomena are prominent in ordinary characterizations of health and ill-health: 1) certain kinds of feelings — that is, feelings of well-being and ease when we speak of health and feelings of suffering and pain when we speak of ill-health, and 2) the phenomena of ability (in the case of health) and disability (in the case of ill-health). Nordenfelt opts for ability/disability as the more central kind of phenomena and founds his analysis of health on the concept of ability. In accord with Pörn he distinguishes between opportunities to act and abilities to act, the former referring to external, situational factors and the latter to the internal set-up of the person. This makes it possible to characterize the meaning of "ability to act" in a more precise manner. To say of a person that he has the ability to perform a certain act, does not mean to say that he performs the act if he tries (since the opportunities may be lacking), and it does not mean to say that he performs the act under some circumstances if he tries (since there could be extremely advantageous circumstances that would allow him to perform the act even if his internal set-up were extremely poor). What we mean, Nordenfelt suggests, by saying that a person has the ability to act in a certain way, is that he will actually perform the act if he tries, under standard circumstances. What are standard circumstances? This, of course, is a matter of definition by choice. Standard circumstances may, and will, vary from one societal context to another, and from one individual to another.

Nordenfelt then introduces a distinction between first-order (actual) ability and second-order (potential) ability. First-order ability means precisely the ability to perform an act, if one tries, under standard circumstances. Second-order ability means a first-order ability to train oneself in order to acquire a first-order ability to perform an act.

From this Nordenfelt can now take a first step towards characterizing health in terms of ability. A person is said to be in a state of health if he has, at least, the second-order ability, given standard circumstances, to perform those acts which are necessary and jointly sufficient for reaching his vital goals. What, then, should be counted as vital goals? The key notion, Nordenfelt proposes, should be the notion of happiness, understood in a general sense, covering such notions as contentedness, satisfaction and pleasure. The vital goals of a person are those states of affairs that he must achieve to be happy. This is then qualified by stating that some degree of minimal happiness (as opposed to complete happiness) is intended, and that long-term happiness (as opposed to momentary happiness) is the notion suggested. So health could now be characterized thus: A person is in a state of health if he is able to reach the states of affairs which are necessary and jointly sufficient for his minimal long-term happiness. Is this characterization value-free or evaluative? It is evaluative in the sense that a decision must be made as to what constitutes minimal happiness.

Against this background the concept of disease can now be defined. A disease is such a phenomenon, internal to a person's body or mind, as tends to compromise his health — that is, tends to cause disability with respect to at least one of his vital goals.

This will have to do as a review of the three theories here chosen to exemplify MMM-inclined reasoning. Obviously the three have very much in common. And perhaps my way of reviewing them has overstressed the similarities. There are also some major differences, especially as regards Nordenfelt's theory as compared with those of Pörn and Whitbeck. Those differences, however, will not be vital when it comes to discussing medical-model conceptions of abnormal behaviour and mental afflictions.

Let me briefly summarize the common features of the three theories. Most important to notice is the taking of the concept of health as the more basic and primary. Also prominent is the placing of the health-analysis in a social, rather than in a biological context. It is the person who is, or is not, in a state of health, rather than some part of his body. The notion of ability plays a crucial role in arriving at a characterization of health, and ability here applies to persons, not to organs or organ-systems. Diseases are defined in terms of their tendency to weaken the abilities of a person vis-à-vis his goals (the goals, in turn, being specified with varying degrees of precision in the different theories). Health is certainly a value-laden notion in these theories. Disease, not being the opposite of health, is all the same value-laden, at least in the sense that an instance of disease earns its status as disease from its tendency to compromise something that has a positive value (health). Disease is distinguished in all three theories from illness, the latter being here, as far as I can see, synonymous with ill-health.

Finally let me briefly sum up the main differences between the two groups of theories, and at the same time recapitulate the distinguishing criteria of the TMM and the MMM, respectively. Obviously there is a major difference between the two sets of theories as regards focusing on the "cause-side" or the "effect-side" of the health-disease complex. Boorse and Ross, by opting for 'disease' as the primary, or more basic, concept actually define ill-health in terms of its causes — that is, in terms of the nature of the "machine-fault" (the statistically abnormal sub-species-typical functioning of some "machine-part") that is the disease. Pörn, Whitbeck and Nordenfelt, by opting for 'health' as the basic concept actually define disease in terms of its effects, or consequences, on a whole-person level, that is in terms of ill-health.

Boorse and Ross clearly belong on a reductionist platform, expressing the nature of higher-level phenomena (health and ill-health) in terms of absence or presence of lower-level phenomena (diseases), while Pörn, Whitbeck and Nordenfelt are holistic in their approach. Health and disease are opposites with Boorse and Ross, while health is something more than absence of disease with Pörn, Whitbeck and Nordenfelt. On the question of values, finally, Boorse and Ross propose the disease-notion to be value-free. Health, in its opposite-of-disease sense, is equally value-free, while 'illness' according to Boorse is value-laden. Pörn, Whitbeck and Nordenfelt propose 'health' to be evaluative, while remaining a bit more unclear as to the value-status of 'disease', though the fact that disease is defined in terms of its compromising effects on health makes it seem plausible to suggest that some value-dimension pertains to the disease-concept also.

On distinguishing illness from disease

Now, the outline of some TMM- and MMM-inclined theories has left us with some ambiguities as to meanings of key terms, and these need addressing before we can move on to a substantial retesting of the strength of the critique of the notion of mental illness.

A source of much confusion in the debate on mental illness, I believe, is the fact that "illness" and "disease" by some writers are used as synonymous expressions, whereas others make a distinction of meaning between the two. Szasz belongs to the former and so do many of his opponents. The distinguishing of "disease" from "illness" seems to some extent to be part of the development of medical-philosophical theorizing that has taken place primarily after the period when "anti-psychiatric" criticism was most intense. In the writings of those defending psychiatry during the late 1960's and early 70's one does not find much arguing that takes issue on this distinction. I believe that it is a pertinent remark in this context to say that the interchangeable (synonym-) use of "illness" and "disease" is not "faulty". There *is* a usage where these terms function as synonyms. Consulting a dictionary will support this.[16] "To suffer from a disease" and "to suffer from an illness" could certainly be said to express the same thing.

Through the first two chapters of this study "disease" and "illness" have been used interchangeably in accordance with the usage of Szasz and other writers referred to. The disease-illness distinctions proposed by the writers reviewed in this chapter now force us to abandon this assumption of synonymity. How, then, should "disease" and "illness" be distinguished? This is not self-evident, since different writers tend to make the distinction in different ways. I shall give a few examples. One, quite early, suggestion of how to make the distinction was made by Feinstein.[17] He proposes that "disease" should denote the underlying organic abnormality that is at the root of the problems that force a person to see a doctor. A description of a disease is in terms of morphologic, physiological, chemical, micro-biological etc. variables, telling us something about the structure or function of the organism, or some part of it, of the patient. The "illness" of the same patient, on the other hand, according to Feinstein, is the clinical manifestation of the disease (the disease being, more often than not, detectable only in the laboratory or in the autopsyroom). The illness, in Feinstein's view, consists of signs, that the doctor detects during his examination, and symptoms, that the patient experiences.

Reading[18] suggests a distinction that is partly analogous. "Disease" refers, according to him, to the structural disorder of tissues and organs that constitutes the organic abnormality of the diseased person. "Illness" denotes the experiences of the diseased person; his pain and discomfort, his suffering and incapacitation. Reading literally speaks of these as separate entities, that can exist quite independently of each other.

A third suggestion is made by Fitzpatrick,[19] who proposes that "illness" refers to the subjective interpretation of problems which are perceived to be health-related, while "disease" refers to a medical conception of pathological abnormality diagnosed by means of signs and symptoms.

Now the disease-illness distinctions made by the theorists reviewed earlier in this chapter partly reflect and partly diverge from the just mentioned ones. To Boorse "disease" refers to the statistically abnormal subpar functioning of some part of the organism of a person. "Illness", in his scheme, seems to denote, not a consequence or an effect of the disease with regard to the experiential or global level of the person carrying the disease, but rather a sub-class of disease, viz. the one containing the diseases that are incapacitating and therefore treatment-deserving, and that constitute grounds for the removal of moral blame. It is not the case, in Boorse's theory, that there are two "things" or entities, the disease and the illness. Illnesses are diseases of a certain kind and diseases are illnesses that lack some dimensions or attributes.

Nordenfelt, Pörn and Whitbeck seem to view illness as something quite different. The requirements of something being viewed as an illness-instance on their terms are, as far as I can see, primarily that incapacitation of a person is at hand and that the cause of the incapacitation is internal. There is no requirement of the presence of a disease for it being pertinent to call somebody ill.

The same diversity of expression applies, as we have seen, to the use of the term health and to the proposed relations between the concept of health and the concepts of disease and illness. To Boorse health is the opposite of disease. To Nordenfelt, Pörn and Whitbeck health is the opposite of illness.

These differences are interesting and important from the point of view of this study for several reasons. They tell us something about the state of ambiguity and uncertainty that characterizes the discussion of the health-disease concept complex in general. And, which is more to the point, they make the discussion of the critique of the medical-model conception of so-called mental-illness phenomena somewhat problematic. It would seem that we can no longer be certain exactly what it is that the critique is directed against, or what it is that various defenders of the medical-model conception actually defend. To be able to take the discussion some steps further, we shall have to make some stipulations. I shall, from here on, take it as evident that the thrust of the Szaszian type of critique, with regard to its more theoretical dimensions, of the concept of mental illness is intended primarily to question the notion of *mental disease*. It is the claim that "mental illnesses" are disease-type problems, on a par with somatic or "ordinary" disease-type problems and satisfying the disease-status criteria of those problems, that the critique, at its heart, is directed against. This means that the concept of mental disease should be the focus of our attention for much of the discussion to follow.

Notes

1 Ludwig, A. M.: The Psychiatrist as Physician, in *Journal of the American Medical Association*, 234, 6, 1975, pp. 603-604.
2 Ibid. p. 603.
3 Engel, G. L.: The Need for a New Medical Model, in Caplan, A. L., Engelhardt, H. T., Jr. and McCartney, J. J. (eds.): *Concepts of Health and Disease*.
4 Ibid.
5 Ibid. p. 595.
6 Ibid. p. 598.
7 Boorse, C.: Health as a Theoretical Concept, in *Philosophy of Science*, 44, 1977, pp. 542-573, and On the Distinction between Disease and Illness.
8 Ross, A.: Sygdomsbegrebet, *in Bibliotek for laeger*, 171, 2, 1979. pp. 111-129.
9 Boorse, C.: Health as a Theoretical Concept, p. 556.
10 Boorse, C: On the Distinction Between Disease and Illness, p. 61.
11 Pörn, I.: An Equilibrium Model of Health, in Nordenfelt, L. and Lindahl, B. I. B. (eds.).: *Health, Disease and Causal Explanation in Medicine*, Dordrecht, 1984.
12 Whitbeck, C.: A Theory of Health, in Caplan, A. L., Engelhardt, H. T., Jr. and McCartney, J. J. (eds.): *Concepts of Health and Disease*.
13 Ibid. p. 611.
14 Ibid. p. 611.
15 Nordenfelt, L.: *On the Nature of Health. An Action-Theoretic Approach*, Dordrecht, 1987.
16 See, for instance, *Oxford Advanced Learner's Dictionary of Current English* (A.S. Hornby, ed.), eighth impression, Oxford, 1978.
17 Feinstein, A.: *Clinical Judgement*, Baltimore, 1967.
18 Reading, A.: Illness and Disease, in *Medical Clinics of North America*, 61, 4, 1979, pp. 703-710.

19 Fitzpatrick, R. M.: Social Concepts of Illness and Disease, in Patrick, D. L. and Scambler, G. (eds.): *Sociology as Applied to Medicine*, London, 1982.

5 Disease in general and "mental disease"

Introductory notes

We thus have made a basis for trying to take the discussion of the criticism of the medical-model conception of abnormal behaviour and mental afflictions some steps further. I have distinguished, and outlined in ideal-type form, two medical models, with the purpose of helping to articulate some explicit and implicit notions underpinning the objections to the Szaszian position. I have reviewed a number of TMM-inclined and MMM-inclined theories of health and disease, with the intention of substantiating the ideal-type constructions and reflecting some medical-philosophical development having taken place since the time of the most intense flourishing of the criticism of the notion of mental illness. And I have somewhat elaborated upon the various suggestions of relations between the notions of health, disease and illness, and stipulated that the notion of mental disease should be the one focused on.

I shall now move on to a renewed attempt at assessing the strength of the Szaszian type of critique. I shall concentrate on three issues, that I take to be the crucial ones in trying to advance the analysis. The first, and probably the most important, issue concerns the divergence of foci, on the "cause-side" (within TMM-reasoning) or on the "effect-side" (within MMM-reasoning) of the disease-health complex, when trying to apply medical-model reasoning to abnormal behaviour and mental afflictions. The second issue has to do with the importance of different stands on the question of value-components of disease-status decisions, when discussing analogies and disanalogies between "ordinary" and "mental" diseases. The third issue, that will play a somewhat less important role in the discussion, concerns the relations between the concepts of disease, illness and health in the context of the discussion. These issues will tend to overlap and become intermingled to some extent. Towards the end of the chapter, however, I shall try to disentangle them, and summarize the outcome of the discussion with regard to each one of them separately.

At this point I would like to recall and restate a presupposition of medical-model reasoning that I discussed briefly in chapter 1, and that I take to be crucial to the discussion. A medical-model view of so-called mental-illness phenomena implies claiming that there are two sub-categories of diseases: bodily diseases and mental diseases. The "mental diseases" are supposed, on the one hand to be relevantly *dissimilar* to bodily diseases for the distinction between the two sub-categories of diseases to be meaningful, and on the other hand to be relevantly *similar* to bodily diseases for the two categories to be reasonably subsumed under a common head-category of disease. This requirement of a similarity of "mental diseases" to bodily diseases is also expressed in my first postulate (page 11) as a condition of the reasonableness of conceptualizing the former phenomena in terms of disease. It is important that we keep this in mind as we move along.

Now one important distinction is between notions of abnormal behaviour and mental afflictions as *signs* and/or *symptoms* of "mental disease" and as *constitutive* of "mental disease". As we saw in chapter 3, discussing Ausubel's objections to Szasz's critique, the latter view is preferred by some writers. This view, however, implies a substantial step away from common medical-model reasoning, in that it entails abandoning the disease/disease-sign/disease-symptom separating that is central to discourse on "ordinary" disease. This view therefore undoubtedly will involve severe problems when it comes to arguing for the adequacy of the medical-model conception of abnormal behaviour and mental afflictions. It also seems to entail some very problematic aspects when it comes to distinguishing abnormal behaviour that is disease from abnormal behaviour that is non-disease. I believe that this view could only retain the medical-model conception by way of some or other form of metaphor-reasoning.

The view that abnormal behaviour and mental afflictions are signs and/or symptoms of "mental disease" obviously keeps up a greater closeness to ordinary medical-model reasoning. The notion is here that "mental disease" itself is some pathological phenomenon residing within the person who behaves abnormally. This view provides the basis for a fundamentalist notion of the reasonableness of conceptualizing abnormal behaviour and mental afflictions in terms of "mental disease". And it is against this notion that we shall take the Szaszian type of critique to be primarily directed. Two questions seem immediately to present themselves. What is the nature of the internal pathology that produces the signs and symptoms of "mental disease" — that is, of the "mental disease" itself? And, most important, in what sense is this pathology of the same nature as the pathology ordinarily (that is, in undisputed instances of bodily disease) called disease? The discussions to follow will, to a substantial degree, be centred around different answers to these two questions.

The Szaszian type of critique is heavily founded on the claim that a necessary condition of disease is the presence of a certain type of abnormality, internal to the organism of the diseased individual. And Szasz claims further that this internal abnormality, for it to be appropriately spoken of as disease, should be an *organic* abnormality (a "machine-fault") causing the problems of the afflicted individual. Therefore, says Szasz, there could be no such thing as a "mental disease". Following the various notions of disease expressed by adherents of TMM- and MMM-inclined theories of health and disease, we could now distinguish two ways to meet this criticism. We could either try to argue, on the platform of the TMM, that there *are* in "mental disease" pathological internal abnormalities present, analogous to the ones present in "ordinary" disease, causing the behavioural and/or experiental signs or symptoms. Or we could try to argue, on an MMM platform, that there is no requirement of a certain type of internal cause, for it being appropriate to speak of disease, since 'disease' is defined in terms of the *effects* of internal factors on the capacity-level of a person.

The TMM approach

Let us turn to the TMM platform for the defence first. There seem to be two versions of the TMM-inclined defence. There is the view that the internal pathology in cases of "mental disease" is of *exactly* the same type as in cases of physical disease, which is to say that "mental disease" pathology, just like other pathology, is assumed to consist of structural or functional abnormalities of the human organism. This is the somaticist view of "mental disease". But it could also, on the TMM platform, be argued that the internal abnormalities in cases of "mental disease" are not, and need not be, of an organic nature for them to be correctly conceptualized in terms of disease. What is required is that they satisfy the criteria of disease, which are expressed in terms of deviations from norms of functioning. This is a defence of a notion of "mental disease" *sui generis*, purely mental disease.

The somaticist TMM approach

Let us tackle the somaticist view first. This is the view of many biologically oriented psychiatric theorists. For several reasons I believe that this approach is ill-suited to defending the concept of mental disease. The main problem is to adequately answer the question of how, and why, "mental disease" should be distinguished from physical disease on this view. If the disease that causes behavioural or experiential abnormalities is organic by nature, what is mental about it? There is a choice of distinguishing "mental disease" from bodily disease either by way of pointing to different causes of human ailments or by way of pointing to different effects of internal abnormalities. The cause-differentiating approach has been openly rejected by upholders of the somaticist view. Remains the effect-differentiating approach. But this will run into problems inasmuch as many well-established bodily diseases have mainly psychological or behavioural consequences for the patient. Diverse conditions of the brain, like tumours or haemhorrages, are not regarded as mental diseases. And a large part of what are considered unequivocally bodily diseases (ranging from malaria to an inflamed tooth) would, with this view, have to be considered at least partly mental. And contrariwise, many diseases now considered to be "mental diseases" have in fact largely bodily effects or consequences. Conversion hysteria is perhaps the best example of this.

The key problem, it seems, with the somaticist view of "mental disease" is that it, instead of firmly establishing "mental disease" as a sub-category of disease on a par with bodily disease, runs the risk of making the notion of mental disease redundant. "Mental disease" with this view seems to be reduced to physical disease. By insisting on a physical basis of mental afflictions and behavioural disturbances one has let go of the possibility of stating the criteria by which to distinguish the two sub-categories of disease ("mental" and somatic). Now observe that this problematization of the somaticist view does not imply subscribing to the notion that the phenomena called mental diseases should have no physical bases. On the contrary it is in accord with the supposition that all human behaviour and experience have some biological bases. The problem is rather that to distinguish "non-diseased" behaviour from "diseased" behaviour we could not point to the diseased or non-diseased nature of the *biological* basis of the behaviour. Because that would lead us exactly to reducing "mental disease" to physical disease. The "mental disease" would be a consequence or effect of physical disease. But to retain the notion of mental disease we would rather have to avoid pointing to physical disease as its basis. That is, the pathology of the mental state or the behavioural display that we would like to call "diseased" must be located somewhere else than in the biological basis of the state or behaviour.

I shall try to formulate the problematic aspect of the somaticist view of "mental disease" in another way to make the point clear. Obviously people have been classified as "mentally diseased" for a very long time, during the whole course of psychiatry's existence as a medical-scientific discipline, despite the failure to find organic abnormalities underpinning the classification. And this has been done either because the view has been held that physical pathology is not a requirement of disease, or because the view has been held that physical pathology will eventually and in the course of scientific development and research be discovered and shown to account for the "diseased" behaviours and mental conditions — the latter view being the somaticist one. This latter view implies that the notion of a disease-nature of "mental diseases" is really taken to hinge on the existence of physical abnormality (yet to be discovered) in the persons spoken of as "mentally diseased". If one did not believe in the existence of such abnormalities, one would not, with this view, agree that the persons in question were diseased. Now, let us on the grounds of this description of the somaticist view make some thought-experiments. Suppose that it becomes possible to correlate physical abnormalities, let us say some bio-chemical abnormalities of the brain, with behavioural abnormalities to a far greater extent than is now possible. And suppose that a number of persons deemed "mentally diseased", displaying very similar behaviour and mental conditions, were found to harbour *different* bio-chemical abnormalities. From the somaticist point of view, would we say that they were suffering from different diseases that showed similar symptoms, or would we say that they suffered from the same disease which could have different physical correlates? If we were to choose the second interpretation, we would seem to have admitted that the "disease" is the symptom-cluster rather than its cause, which seems incompatible with the somaticist premises. If we opted for the first interpretation, which I believe we ought to on the somaticist premises, this would undoubtedly entail remaking the classification system of "mental diseases" that is now with us, since this is based on symptomatological features — but this need not bother us in this context. The point, so far, is just that the experiment highlights the consequences of tying the stating of disease-nature and the distinguishing among diseases in instances of "mental disease" to the physical abnormality assumed to constitute its biological base (and not to its consequences). Now suppose that we found some people harbouring the bio-chemical abnormality that was assumed to be responsible for the disturbed behaviour of some of the "mentally diseased" persons mentioned above, but that these persons did *not* display the disturbed behaviour. Would the defender of the somaticist position on "mental disease" not have to say that these persons were "mentally diseased"? I think he would. That is, you could not declare these normal-functioning persons not to be "mentally diseased" on account of their lack of behavioural symptoms of "mental disease", and at the same time deem behavioural symptoms irrelevant to the decision as to which "mental disease" people with diverse bio-chemical abnormalities are to have ascribed to them. Either the nature of a person's behaviour and of his mental state is relevant to decisions regarding his disease-state or it is not. So the symptom-free person with the bio-chemical abnormality would be "mentally diseased", just as a person with a cancer tumour in his tissues would be said to suffer from cancer even if no symptom-level phenomena had evolved. And this, to finally come to the point of this thought-experiment, would make it perfectly clear that "mental disease" is *nothing* but physical disease, and that there is *nothing* mental whatsoever about the disease-nature of "mental disease" on the somaticist position.

The genuine-mental-disease TMM approach

Now let us turn to the second type of defence of a notion of mental disease, within TMM-inclined reasoning, which I believe to be superior to the somaticist type, from the point of view of logic and reasonableness, but which is, as we shall see, not without problems. The key notion here is that the internal pathology of the "mentally diseased" is not located in the organic, but in the psychic, apparatus. We are invited to take the step into a kind of medical discourse where, if there is a "machine-fault", it is the *psychic* machinery, not the organic, that has broken down. And, according to this approach, the notion of disease is equally applicable in discourses on psychic dysfunctional abnormalities as is the case when we speak of somatic pathology. The phenomena called mental diseases, it is claimed, can be shown to satisfy the same criteria of disease that apply in somatic medicine.

It must be noted here that Szasz and many other critics would probably claim that talk of a "psychic apparatus" is purely metaphorical. And to some extent I am inclined to agree. The mind "is" not a machine. It is possible, of course, to talk of the mind, or psyche, *as if* it was an apparatus. This is to lay the metaphor open. But, it could be argued, why should we want to use this metaphorical language? It is not self-evident that this is a valid, or even fruitful, way of characterizing, and providing with a context, the phenomena called mental. And it is even less evident that it provides us with a reasonable conceptual framwork for discussing the nature of the phenomena called "mental diseases". Let us remember that the "machine-model" talk of the human organism is itself metaphorical. It does not imply believing that the human body is a machine. But in the case of the body one can readily acknowledge the fruitfulness of the metaphor. It helps us, to some extent, to grasp some aspects of the nature of the workings of the interlocking functional systems that sustain the life-processes of the organism. But why extend this metaphor to the psyche or mind? It is as if we were being asked to picture a machine within a machine, which seems a bit strange. So one straight-forward reaction to the extension of the functional-system-disturbance view of bodily disease to include "mental disease" would be to flatly reject the step we are invited to take.

But this, of course, would be premature as well as unfair. There might be some striking similarities between "ordinary" diseases and "mental diseases" that we are able to recognize only after tentatively agreeing that "mental functional systems" could plausibly be regarded as analogous in some respects to bodily organs, and that the "mental apparatus" is a plausible analogue to the multi-functional system of an organism as a whole. And maybe we could even be convinced that mental entities could malfunction in a way that allows for the application of the term "disease" to that malfunctioning.

To approach an understanding of the way mental phenomena could be viewed as diseases in analogy with bodily diseases, we could start by making a list of bodily functional systems that could be thought of as possible seats of disease. Such a list would include entities like the heart, the lungs, the kidneys, the skin, etc. And the brain would certainly have a place in this list. But suppose we should add "the mind" to the list. This would seem to be a mistake. "The mind" is not an entity of the same kind as the other items on the list. Those are parts of the body — which, of course, is why diseases of any one of them will be included under the heading of "physical diseases". But the mind belongs to another category of phenomena. If we want to show that diseases can pertain to the mind, as well as (and even in the same sense as) to the body, we would rather have to make two separate lists of possible seats of disease: list number one, comprising heart, lungs, etc., or, more abstractly, bodily functional system 1, bodily functional system 2.....bodily functional system n; and list number two, comprising mental functional system 1, mental functional system 2.....mental functional system n. We would then proceed to show that disease is a type of phenomenon that could be said to apply to the list number-one type of phenomena and the list number-two type of phenomena in exactly the same sense. Now, with this outline of the issue, a number of problems for the defender of a category of genuine "mental diseases" seem to present themselves immediately. To begin with, this separating of bodily and mental functional systems, both types being possible seats of disease, seems to be an expression of a dualist position on the question of the relation of mind to body. And since mind-body dualism is nowadays rather a discredited position within the philosophy of mind (not to mention its status within medical science) it would seem preferable to avoid it. This implies sticking to the notion that all mental phenomena are somehow correlated with physical, or bodily, phenomena. So a mental functional system would have to be thought of as based in the organism of the individual. But, granted that this is so, it seems close at hand to suppose that a "diseased" mental functional system must have its base in a diseased part of the organism. That is, if normal mental functioning is correlated with normal biological functioning of the brain, it would seem plausible that a malfunctioning mental system is correlated with a malfunctioning brain (or part of the brain). But this would throw us back on the somaticist position. It would imply viewing "mental disease" as an outcome of, or a consequence of, bodily disease. And this, of course, is exactly what the defender of genuine "mental disease" must avoid, since it would render the notion of mental disease redundant. So, the dilemma here seems to be to avoid the dualist mind-body position while still retaining the notion of separate mental functions being not directly related to bodily (cerebral) functions that could be specifically tied to them.

There is, however, a way out of this dilemma, and Boorse[1] has utilized it fully in his defence of a notion of mental disease separable from, and analogous to, the notion of bodily disease. The argument goes as follows. To agree that every mental event is correlated with a physical event does not entail agreeing that every *type* of mental event is correlated with a type of physical events. That a certain mental condition (say, to use Boorse's example, a desire for a lobster dinner) is present in a person does not imply that a certain type of physical condition is present in every person that holds the same mental condition. Different neural configurations in different people could play the same motivational role. Therefore "there may be no set of anatomical properties that could define the mentalistic term 'desire for a lobster dinner'; the mentalistic vocabulary, even for a materialist, may not be neurologically definable".[2] And this actually, says Boorse, is why rejecting dualism does not entail destroying the autonomy of psychiatry as a discipline with an area of expertise of its own. A disease-type defined in mentalistic terms can not be presupposed to coincide with a disease-type defined in physiological terms. There may not be any distinctive neural similarity between the brains of patients who have the same "mental disease". Therefore "mental diseases" may fail to be physical diseases, since they cannot be defined in physiological terms. "If the mentalistic vocabulary is not neurologically definable, there will be no way to reduce causal laws of the mind to causal laws of the body."[3] Therefore "mental diseases" will typically be explained in mental causal terms, not in physical causal terms. An explanation of a "mental disease" will be in terms of feelings, beliefs and experiences, not in terms of physiological variables. So a non-dualist view of mind-body relations is, it would seem, after all compatible with not reverting to a somaticist view of "mental disease".

Now, we would have to agree with Boorse that he has found a way out of the dilemma outlined above. Observe, however, that there is some degree of hypothetical reasoning in "the Boorsian escape". His case seems to rest on premises that are title to some doubt, or at least some caution. We should note that this defence of the reasonableness of a concept of mental disease is built on the probability of the correctness of a certain type of identity-theory on the issue of mind-body relations. There are a lot of "this-may-be-so's" in the argument he presents. Should this theory of mind-body relations turn out to be invalid, for instance due to successful research along somaticist lines, the Boorsian genuine-mental-disease defence would seem to collapse. We should also note that if physical *types* of events could eventually be correlated with "mental-disease" *types* of events in some instances of "mental disease", those "mental diseases" would stop being mental diseases, on the Boorsian position.

Observe also that the Boorsian solution leaves us with an obvious disanalogy between bodily and "mental" diseases. If we compare the two lists of functional systems, the bodily and the mental, and reflect upon the characteristics of possible diseases of different items on the lists, we cannot escape noting one obvious dissimilarity between items on the "body-list" and items on the "mind-list". A bodily functional system, let us say an organ, is diseased on the TMM view when it functions sub-par. But a prominent characteristic of the overwhelming majority of bodily diseases is also that this reduced function is due to a *structural* abnormality. Typically the malfunctioning of a lung, or a kidney, is caused by an alteration in structure that prevents the organ from functioning normally. It stretches the imagination to see how a disturbance of a mental function could be seen as analogously structurally caused. Now, there are certainly instances of bodily malfunctioning where structural abnormalities have not been detected. In these cases one tends to speak of "functional diseases" of the body. Typically, however, this does not imply that there *are* no structural abnormalities connected to the disease in question. The notion is rather that the structural abnormality component of the disease escapes our present state of knowledge and that the disease in question is therefore insufficiently described and explained. In "mental disease"-type malfunctionings there could be no structural abnormality on the Boorsian premises. A "mental disease" related structural abnormality would have to be looked for either in the biological basis of the mental function deemed to be diseased, which would turn us back on the somaticist approach and imply the reduction of "mental disease" to physical disease, or in the "mind" itself which would of course imply the most absurd kind of mind-body dualism. So the avoiding of mind-body dualism and physical reductionism leaves us with at least one prominent disanalogy between the set of characteristics of bodily diseases and those of "mental diseases" on the genuine-mental-disease version of the TMM approach.

But let us pursue the discussion on the premises that the dilemmas of mind-body dualism and somaticist reductionism have been successfully dealt with. We can now begin to tackle the key notions of this TMM version of the defence of the concept of mental disease. The credibility of analogous reasoning, on matters of disease and health, in the bodily and the mental areas of discourse, rests, I believe, on two or three crucial points. The first one is the need of demonstrating that there are mental functions that are, in relevant aspects, analogous to bodily functions. The second is the need to show that those functions can be spoken of as normal and abnormal in the same sense that we (according to Boorse and Ross) speak of bodily functions. And the third, which is closely connected to the second, is the necessity of demonstrating that the value-neutrality that (according to Boorse and Ross) pertains to bodily-disease decisions is equally at work in typical instances of "mental disease" decisions.

Let me briefly recapitulate the features of a TMM notion of bodily disease. Such a disease is said to be present when some part of the body fails to perform its, statistically establishable, species-typical contribution to the life-processes of the organism. This sub-par functioning is a matter of objective statement of facts, and the ascription of disease is not a matter of evaluation. There is a "natural order", a plan of organisation developed through natural evolution, of the human organism, and diseases are deviations from this "species-design". So the notions of natural function and statistical normality are corner-stones of this medical model. But there are other notions of, or senses of, functioning and normality that could be distinguished from those utilized in the TMM. When we speak of a person's co-existence with, and interactions with, his social environment, we could speak of "social functioning". This social functioning would then differ from biological functioning in some important respects. There would be no "design", objectively detectable, for the social kind of functioning. On the contrary, an important characteristic of social life is its tremendous flexibility and diversity as to forms and organisational features, it could be argued. And when we speak of normality and abnormality in the context of social functioning, there is no intimation of deviance from a "natural" (in the biological sense) order or plan. So normality in a social sense, seems to differ from normality in the biological sense. One way to express the difference is to distinguish between statistical normality and normative normality, the former being a straightforward matter of empirical investigation, and the latter being an evaluative choice of what should be deemed desirable. An important question to put now to TMM spokesmen, like Boorse, is this one: Can it be shown that assessments of mental normal-functioning, and the deviations from it called mental diseases, are matters of decisions of the natural-function (biological, statistical, non-evaluative) kind and not of the social (normative, evaluative) kind of normality? Because to the extent that the latter kind of normality decisions should enter into ascriptions of "mental" health and disease, to the same extent would the TMM-version of the medical-model conception of abnormal behaviour and mental afflictions lose its validity.

What is a "mental function" that could be viewed as analogous to a bodily function, for instance that of an organ? This is not self-evident. According to Boorse[4] mental disease is explained, not in terms of physiological factors, but in terms of beliefs, feelings and experiences. Are these mental functions? I shall attempt a discussion in two steps. First I shall discuss the possibility of ascribing disease-status to the just mentioned kind of mental phenomena, and then I shall go on to discuss in general and broad terms a more elaborate and specific approach to what it is about the mental that can be viewed as diseased. For the first part of this discussion I shall rely, to some extent, on de Sousa,[5] who has analyzed the notion of normality as applied to beliefs, desires and experiences, which he takes to be the broadest categories of mental functions. De Sousa's discussion is not directed at Boorse, but I think some of his insights could be utilized to counter Boorse's position.

One of the most common traits of persons deemed to be "mentally diseased" is that they hold *beliefs* that are judged to be strange and uncalled-for. Could it be the case that there is a mental function, "the belief function", that could be sub-par functioning as matched against the species design? We should note, however, that not all kinds of abnormal beliefs are deemed "mentally diseased". A ready-at-hand exception is the case of the religious fanatic. Members of various religious sects are known to hold beliefs, and hold them with a fervour and intensity that well matches that of the schizophrenic paranoiac, that are wildly at odds with the majority view. It seems that what saves the members of such sects from being labelled insane or "mentally diseased" is precisely that they are members — that is, parties to a shared view of reality. If this is so, an interesting question is how small a number of sect-members we should allow to hold a particular set of fantastic beliefs before we would start questioning their mental health. Or, to turn the issue around: If a psychotic person succeeded in converting some fellow human beings to his interpretation of reality, and they formed a sect together, would he then stop being "mentally diseased"? Or would the others turn psychotic? It seems obvious from these considerations that we will run into counter-intuitive considerations when we try to base the disease-nature of beliefs on statistical infrequency. The infrequency of holding a set of beliefs could not be what really determines the "mentally diseased" status of the harbourer of the beliefs. Nor does it seem to be the degree of falsity or absurdity of the beliefs, from the majority point of view, that provides the basis of the disease-decision. So where is this basis? One way to answer this could be to claim that holding belief-systems that people are *socialized* into holding, or belief-systems that are already *there* and that one chooses to accept, does not express diseased belief-functioning. It is the production of a belief-system that is at odds with the majority view, from "within", that points to such disease. This would, however, leave the founders of religious sects, or the constructors of great religious systems, in the diseased category, which would seem to be a less than welcome solution from the followers' point of view.

This comparing of psychotic belief-systems to religious belief-systems might seem provocative and out of place, but I believe that it is important to make clear the implications. A striking dissimilarity between the odd belief-system of a person deemed "mentally diseased" and that of a member of a religious minority, is that the latter shows some degree of conformity in believing, albeit it is not a conformity to the belief-system of a majority, while the former shows a complete lack of conformity to current belief-systems in the person's social milieu. Should this be the real distinguishing criterion of a diseased belief-function, however, it would seem that we have crossed the line into social-evaluative normality-assessments, since requirements of conformity to prevalent belief-systems could not reasonably be thought of as having to do with scientific, objective statement of facts.

But let us try another approach to the "belief-function" as a candidate for being a mental entity that could be viewed as diseased. De Sousa points out that beliefs ought not only to be reasonably true, but that we ought to *arrive* at them in a certain way. The "disturbance" of the belief-function might consist in a faulty way of acquiring beliefs or of a failure in passing from one belief to another in a certain, correct, way. And it seems that this way of viewing the belief-function disturbance might provide the basis for some analogy with disturbed bodily function, since behaviour is to some extent based on belief, and the acquirement of reasonably true beliefs might therefore prove important to survival. This means requiring that the forming of beliefs, for it to be seen as normal-functioning, should adhere to standards of why and how this or that belief ought, or ought not, to be held. The main problem here, writes de Sousa, is that beliefs are not, in most cases, accepted on the basis of evidence or reason at all. The set of beliefs that are dominant in a certain social environment are accepted precisely because they *are* dominant. And, besides, we seem to be back with the religious-fanatic example again. The beliefs most often assessed as "fantastic" or "strange" and most unaccountable for by way of reasoning, logic and evidence, are to be found among mysticists and religious fanatics. We would not apply the disease-scheme to those. We would only regard them as abnormal from the point of view of social and evaluative standards. All this, of course, does not mean to say that we could not distinguish beliefs according to degrees of irrationality, or assess people's greater or lesser adherence to accepted standards of belief-forming. But it means that the notion of normality, when applied to belief, seems to be not of the biological kind, but to rely rather heavily on social and evaluative considerations.

How about desires then? Is it possible to construe abnormality of desires as on a par with sub-par functioning of bodily organs? Somewhat the same problem as with beliefs seems to attach to abnormal desires. The mere statistical infrequency of a particular desire could not be made the basis of disease-ascription. And, most important, the abnormality of desires seems to hold a strong component of the evaluative kind of abnormality. A survey of statistically abnormal desires would be inaccomplishable simply because people would be well aware of which desires to report and which not to if they wanted to appear normal (in the *normative* sense, that is). The norms by which we ordinarily judge desires are, for the most part, explicitly social norms. Generally speaking people could harbour (and probably do) almost any kind of desires without being viewed as abnormal, as long as their acting on the basis of those desires did not throw them into conflict with their social surroundings. And when this occurred it would be more probable than not that a judgement along moral rather than on medical lines would apply. Diverse kinds of sexually abnormal preferences seem to make up the best examples here.

But de Sousa points out that some abnormal desires seem to come closer to the bodily-organ-disorder paradigm. Severe anorexia, the desire to abstain from eating, or a desire for death, an urge to commit suicide, seem to constitute examples of a "disturbed" desire-function, that appears to threaten the preservation of life, in line with disturbances of bodily functions. The objection to the suggestion of an analogy here is provided by de Sousa, who points out that desires differ from bodily diseases in that they can be assessed for rationality. A malfunctioning bodily organ is not an irrational bodily organ. But the concept of rationality is explicitly evaluative, writes de Sousa. That is why "social policy in relation to suicide is a matter of moral decisions".[6] But how about a total absence of desires? Would this not point to a disease-analogous break-down of the desire-function? But, de Sousa notes, the very description of such a condition is made on a theoretical basis. We could choose to interpret the condition in terms of some sort of protest or reaction, and then it would again be subject to assessment of rationality, which brings us back to social and evaluative standards.

Experiences, finally, seem perhaps most difficult to view as "functions" analogous to bodily functions. In most cases of assessing the normality or abnormality of experiences this is closely related to normality-assessments of desires and beliefs. If a person believes that he is the victim of persecution by KGB-agents and suffers agony and depression on account of this, or if he believes that he is one of the chosen few to escape everlasting hell-fire and experiences joy and happiness on account of this, it is the beliefs rather than the experiences that we assess for normality. And those assessments, as we have seen, are heavily intermingled with social and evaluative normality judgements.

But in some instances, such as in manic-depressive conditions, a person may experience severe unhappiness without accompanying "belief- or desire-disturbances" (although these are perhaps, more often than not, also present in such conditions), de Sousa suggests. Here we seem to have a candidate for disturbed "experience-function". But here we have also a type of "mental disease" where the interpretation of the condition typically could diverge into rather distinct and different kinds. On the one hand there are somaticist interpretations, where the "disorder" is viewed as dependent on, and amelioratable by manipulation of, a biological basis of the condition, and on the other hand we have, for instance, social-psychologically oriented interpretations, where the "disorder" is seen as a reaction to environmental factors. In the case of the former view (if it were proven correct) it would be possible to state the decision regarding the disease-status of the condition in value-neutral, matter-of-fact terms (as with regard to any bodily disease on the TMM view). In the case of the latter view it would be possible to make a choice as to whether the abnormality should be said to pertain to the environment or the condition. But to make a case for a genuine-mental-disease view it would have to be stated that the emotion *itself* was diseased. And this would seem to lead us back to rationality asessments again, with the entailed dependence on social and evaluative standards. A psychotic emotion may plausibly be viewed as irrational, but this is not the same as being sub-par functioning in the sense of bodily-organ disease.

The discussion so far has shown, I believe, that there are some problems in assessing beliefs, etc. as diseased in themselves. It seems much more difficult to keep the distinction clear between objectively stated deviations from natural norms and deviations from social-evaluative norms in the realm of mental functionings as compared with the realm of bodily functionings. There are several reasons for this. A main problem seems to be that mental functionings are connected to behaviour, in certain obvious ways that bodily functions are not. It is through assessing a person's behaviour as abnormal that we arrive at assessments of his mental functionings. But this, in turn, causes most discussions of normality and abnormality to become deeply intermingled with social, as opposed to biological, norm systems as standards of assessment.

Consider an important difference between the functioning of an organ and the functioning of an individual in his social environment. While the organ is subject to a quite limited range of possible ways of functioning, if it is to contribute to sustaining the life-processes of the organism, the range of possible ways of social-behavioural functioning is very wide. This, of course, is why Boorse, Ross and others find it possible to speak of species-typical and natural ways of organ-functioning. In many cases a very small alteration of an organ's ways of functioning would turn it into a *dysfunctional* organ, with regard to its species-typical functionings. An individual human being, on the other hand, could be socialized into (and de-socialized out of) a great number of ways of social functioning. This is why a suggestion of a "plan of normality" of social functioning would seem out of place. And this is also why assessments of behaviour in a social context could not rely on objective, value-neutral standards. The norms by which we judge behaviour are social norms, and social norms are explicitly evaluative.

Now, it is this connection to behaviour that creates problems in regarding beliefs, etc. as abnormal in a non-evaluative, natural-biological sense. It is only when we have evaluated the behaviour of an individual as undesirable that we start questioning the normality of the beliefs that would seem to account for the behaviour. And this, I believe, also gives a clue to why the strange beliefs of the religious fanatic do not make us describe his "belief-function" as disordered, while we do describe the beliefs of the psychotic that way. The latter, but not the former, behaves in a way that constitutes severe deviation from some social norm. And this is why the application of the sense of abnormality, that we speak of in cases of disordered organ-functioning, to the mental phenomena discussed above runs into conflict with our knowledge of how "mental diseases" are actually ascribed to people.

All this could now be described as attempts to show a discrepancy between the way *ascriptions* of "mental disease" are actually made, and the way they ought to be made on the TMM premises along the lines suggested by, for instance, Boorse. This would not necessarily imply that Boorse is wrong on theoretical grounds. It would mean though, that Boorse's scheme for delineating "mental disease" is terribly out of touch with the everyday realities of "mental-disease" ascription. This, however, could be taken to suggest a criticism of this reality rather than of Boorse.

An important possible objection to the discussion above must now be articulated and seriously dealt with. It could be argued that the examples of "mental functions" discussed are not really "functions" at all, but rather *products* of such functions. A mental "function", one could suggest, is the "entity" that works to give rise to the phenomena in question. And this brings us to some further considerations of the way "mental disease" is related to behaviour in a sense that differs from the way bodily disease is related to behaviour. "Mental disease", it seems, must always be inferred from behavioural evidence. There is no way to inspect a mental function (or the mind as a whole) to establish the presence of sub-par functioning. It is only through a process of stepwise inference that a decision regarding the "diseased" nature of the mind of a person could be arrived at. This means that the abnormality of a person's mind must be deduced from the abnormality of his behaviour. But in decisions regarding abnormality of behaviour the norm is certainly social rather than biological. It is this inferential step from behavioural (and therefore social, and therefore evaluative) abnormality to mental (biological, species-design-related, non-evaluative) malfunctioning that seems hopelessly untenable. The problem comes clearly into focus if we return for a moment to the somaticist view. Suppose that a specific, bio-chemical, abnormality was beyond any doubt found to cause, to produce, a certain type of behavioural abnormality. When instances of this type of behavioural abnormality occurred in a person, we could always look for evidence of the bio-chemical abnormality in the person, and if it was found we would decide that the person behaved the way he did on account of the bio-chemical abnormality — on account, that is, of a bodily disease. If we did not find the bio-chemical abnormality we would have to state that the person did not suffer from this disease. Either we would then propose that he suffered from some other disease that accounted for his behavioural anomaly, and search for evidence of that, or we would decide that perhaps he was not diseased at all. With the genuine-mental-disease approach we are stuck with the behavioural anomaly, and with no even remotely similar way to validate our disease-hypothesis. What would be required for us to arrive at a disease-decision, in a way analogous to the way decisions regarding physical disease are arrived at, would be a well-established and valid account of the functioning of the human mind, on a par with theories of the functioning of the human body. Not until the coming into being of such a theory of the mind, which would also have to be generally accepted, much like physiological and bio-chemical theories of the workings of the body are accepted by a scientific consensus, would we be able to speak of objectively statable, non-evaluatively normal (in the sense of natural) functions of the mind. *Then* we could approach the question of whether or not these mental functions were such that deviations from normality could be conceived of as satisfying the criteria of disease — the same criteria, that is, that we apply to bodily malfunction. And only if *this* could be shown to be the case would it be pertinent to speak of mental disease in the same sense that we speak of physical disease.

So what we need, really, is a well-established theoretical framework which in descriptive terms tells us what we need to know about the functioning of the human mind. If we turn our attention to the supply of general psychological theories, however, we are faced with a wide spectrum of widely differing basic notions of the human psyche, that seems to offer little promise of providing an encompassing, articulate and univocal account. Within the area of reasoning about "mental health and disease" much the same state of affairs seems to prevail. We could choose to simplify matters by suggesting that two main schools of theory can be roughly distinguished: a behaviouristically inclined and a psycho-analytically inclined. The former would be of little use to us in this context, since it refuses to leave the behavioural level of analysis and has little to tell us of the mind. Psycho-analysis, on the other hand, seems more promising. And psycho-analysis is actually the theoretical framework that Boorse[7] chooses as a platform for articulating his defence of the notion of mental disease.

I shall not, in this context, take it to be my task to discuss the pros and cons of Freudian theory. As everyone knows, it is a theoretical enterprise that is surrounded by much controversy. So, on the point of the requirement of a theory of mind that is univocally accepted as being, at least to a reasonable degree, a correct and encompassing one, psycho-analysis would fall short of the mark. I shall agree with Boorse, however, that it is perhaps the best there is. It is, one could argue, the most well-elaborated and detailed theory of the mental "apparatus". And a whole range of theories of the mind are either superstructures built on the psycho-analytic foundation, or have at least some of the psycho-analytic major assumptions as important premises.

So let us, for the sake of discussion, assess the psycho-analytical theoretical framework of mental functional systems as if it was a univocally accepted and purely (and correctly) descriptive account of the mental area. And the question is, let me repeat this, whether this account of the mental provides a basis for showing that mental functions could be viewed as sub-par functioning, and therefore abnormal, in *the same sense* as this could be the case with diseased bodily functions.

In his brief outline of the relevant features of psycho-analytic theory, Boorse[8] of course takes up the notion of structures of the psyche: the Id, the Ego and the Super-ego. These, he suggests, "could be construed as biological functions".[9] To the Id would be ascribed the motivational function, to the Ego the rationalistic and cognitive function, and to the Super-ego the socialization function. He choses to depart from some Freudian writers who tend to view the gratification of the pleasure-seeking Id as the main function of the Ego, and establishes that the relevancy of speaking of biological functions of the psychic structures rests with their effects on behaviour. Now this, of course, is a very parsimonious sketch of but one of many aspects of Freudian theory. But it is obvious what Boorse is aiming at. Construing these "structures" as biological-functional components of the psychic apparatus opens the door to the possibility of a "species-design" of the mind, and to the possibility of the application of notions of "sub-par functioning" and "mental disease" in a genuine sense.

But the analogy with bodily functions really will not work, and I shall try to show why. The key problem is that the structural view of the psychic apparatus is an explanatory device, that could be utilized to account for *any* way of "functioning". Together with the various other explanatory devices of psycho-analytic theory, such as the conscious-subconscious distinction, the oral-anal-phallic phase development scheme and the cathexis-countercathexis distinction, the structural view will provide a description and explanation of mental functioning accountable for human behaviour and experience. But this account need never be one in terms of *non-functioning*, or "failing" function, in the sense that a diseased bodily function performs sub-par. When the mental structures contribute to the mental functional system as a whole, and ultimately to the behaviour of the individual, in a way that is unacceptable to the individual himself or to his social surroundings, this only means that the *outcome* of one or more of the functional systems is judged to be undesirable. The "function itself" could not be viewed as out of order. The workings, and co-workings, of the mental structures will depend on the life-history of the individual, and especially on important events taking place during the early years of his life. It is important to make as clear as possible this disparity of the ways bodily organs and "mental structures" are viewed as "functioning". Bodily organs have a natural order of functioning built into their very "construction". Either they function well, as matched against this natural order of functioning, or they do not. This is why talk of a species design of bodily functional systems makes sense. A mental functional system will work the way it is "educated" to work, during the period of the individual's life when his mental structures are flexible and shapable. Having acquired its "form" through this "education", it will *function* this way (until the analyst steps into the picture and aids the individual in somewhat "re-educating" it).

This becomes a lot clearer if one takes into account the psycho-analytic view of the development of the individual's mental functioning through early life. It is an important aspect of Freudian theory, from the point of view of the explanation of human character, that the way a child is treated, and the experiences it encounters, will provide clues to the understanding of the character of the grown-up individual. Certain types of events and experiences will tend to produce an "anal" character in the adult (for instance expressed as a fear to "let go" of possessions), while other types of events and experiences will tend to produce an "oral character" (for instance expressed through a tendency to seek oral sensory gratification, as in eating and smoking). These character-differences do not point to the lesser or greater degrees of functioning of one or other mental functional system. They only point to different *ways* of functioning.

To speak of varying degrees of functioning we would have to match the character of the individual against some social standards, which would be culture-specific and relative to societal evaluation systems. Quite a different thing is that in some cases the mental structures of an individual could be "shaped" to produce extremely strange and highly irrational outcomes (beliefs, desires, experiences) which would have behavioural consequences of a dramatic nature. But this would not, this is my contention, point to a break-down of some "natural" (in a biological sense) order of functioning. It would just point to a very *different* way of functioning, and one which would undoubtedly in many cases call for intervention. The point, however, is that the unusual function would not be a disease in the sense that is the case with a cancerous lung that gradually is stopping performing its biologically definable function.

To sum up this appraisal of the "genuine-mental disease" approach on the TMM platform, I think it has been shown that it is somewhat problematic. I have been trying to show that the notions of function, normal-functioning and non-evaluative decisions regarding disease-status are not automatically applicable in the area of mental phenomena. A number of objections could be raised against this application at various stages of analysis, starting with the overall view of the whole enterprise as metaphoric, continuing with various questionings of the reasonableness of trying to ascribe in an objective way disease-status to beliefs, desires, etc., and finally repudiating any similarity between abnormal functionings of mental structural components and abnormal functionings of bodily organs.

We must also take note of the hypothetical moves Boorse, in his account of the reasonableness of a mental-disease notion, is forced to make to arrive at a credible analogy between the bodily and the suggested mental locations of disease. He must found his notion of "pure mental disease" on a certain, by no means validated, theory of mind-body relations; he must choose a theoretical framework of the mental apparatus that is detailed and encompassing enough for interpretations analogous to those regarding the bodily system, but that on exactly this account is controversial and debatable; and he must construe mental functions within this framework "as if" they were analogous to biological functions.[10]

I believe we are justified in remaining sceptical about the possibility of extending to the realm of abnormal behaviour and mental afflictions the theoretical account which is TMM-inclined, has a "cause-side" focus and proposes that disease is a non-evaluative notion.

The MMM approach

So let us turn our attention to the second main alternative for rebutting the Szaszian type of critique of the concept of mental disease on account of the lack of the "right" type of causes in instances of so-called mental disease. This counter-critical strategy will utilize MMM-inclined medical-philosophical theorizing in denying that 'disease' should be defined in terms of a certain type of internal abnormality. It involves arguing instead that the concept of disease is reasonably defined in terms of the effects, or consequences, on the whole-person level of analysis, that internal factors produce.

Now before we turn our attention to a discussion of an MMM-inclined way of arguing for the reasonableness of the mental-disease concept, a few remarks on the strategy of the discussion should be made. I think this is an appropriate place to make clear an implication of the strategy I have chosen for discussing some aspects of different medical models with respect to their applications to abnormal behaviour and mental afflictions. The models (the TMM and the MMM) I have sketched, and the theories I have reviewed as substantiating examples, are obviously very different, and even contradictory, in some respects. This means that both models, and both groups of theories, cannot be accurate in their characterization of health, illness and disease. My strategy, however, entails viewing each model as an existing one (in the theoretical debate at least), and discussing its implications on the premises that it is accurate in its characterization of the notions of "ordinary" health and disease. I have not made it my task to decide *between* the models, or try to assess which one gives a more plausible characterization. This also means that one type of argument that could be used in favour of the Szaszian type of critique is out of reach. I refer to the argument that would follow from analyzing one or other of the medical models and showing it to be incorrect or less satisfying with regard to its success in characterizing the conceptual domain of health and disease.

This strategy of mine obviously also entails a methodologial "flaw", since it could be the case that one of the models seems to provide a reasonable possibility of extending the medical conceptual apparatus to the mental area, and therefore would seem to provide grounds for rejecting the criticism of the concept of mental disease, but that this is made possible through a less correct analysis of the concepts of health and disease in general. Or, contrariwise, if I arrive at the conclusion that one model is not being readily applicable to so-called mental-disease phenomena, this might not be a substantial support of the critical position if the model is inaccurate in its general characterization of health and disease. Short of embarking upon an evaluation of the relative strengths of the two distinct approaches, however (which would lead us into a long and uncertain preliminary analysis), we shall have to accept this drawback to the strategy chosen.

One obvious retort from critics, like Szasz, to a discussion of the reasonableness of a concept of mental disease within an MMM-inclined framework, would be to deny that this sort of framework gives a correct characterization of the general notions of health and disease. It is highly probable that they would claim that characterizations of disease (in general) in terms of incapacitation-tendencies, rather than in terms of the specific internal causes of incapacitation, are out of touch with *the* medical model that is at work within medical science and medico-clinical practice.

Or, even more strongly formulated, it is not improbable that some critics would tend to view this version of the medical model as an ad-hoc construction, suited to legitimizing the medical-model conception of abnormal behaviour and mental afflictions retroactively, *after* it has been adopted for quite non-theoretical reasons. For reasons that will become clear as we move along, I am inclined to agree to some extent with this latter claim, though I hasten to add that this circumstance, from my point of view, probably has nothing to do with the motives of MMM-inclined theorists, but all the more with the methods of conceptual analysis and clarification that they employ.

To go by its face-value the MMM would seem to provide a somewhat better (in the sense of less counter-intuitive) possibility of construing "mental disease" as analogous to bodily disease, than is the case with the TMM. The somaticist reduction of "mental disease" to physical disease, and the problems of showing that mental functions could deviate from a "natural order", that we have discussed in the previous section, would seem to be no hazards to the MMM approach, since disease is here characterized primarily through effects on a whole-person level of analysis. On the face of it this approach would seem to encounter other sorts of problems, such as avoiding an expansion of the disease-concept to include diverse incapacity-producing phenomena that we would maybe not readily accept as diseases. This was the risk facing the various vague notions of disease/illness as suffering and incapacitation, put forward by some of the opponents whose views were discussed in chapter 3. The elaborated MMM-inclined theories, reviewed in chapter 4, that will now serve as a platform for the discussion, are, however, far more exact in their characterization of key notions. We shall see to what extent this makes a difference.

To begin with, the disease-illness distinction would seem to play a far more crucial role for our discussion here than it did for our discussion of the TMM approach. This is due to the different way of making the distinction within each of the two approaches. The Boorsian version of this distinction, it will be remembered, made disease a necessary condition of illness. All instances of illness, with his view, are instances of disease (while not all instances of disease are instances of illness). This made the relations between "mental disease" and "mental illness" unproblematic on the "genuine-disease" view, since "mental illnesses" would be a sub-class of "mental diseases" (provided a class of "mental diseases" could be reasonably delineated). So there would be no problem in keeping "mental disease" related to "mental illness" and bodily disease related to bodily illness while at the same time clearly separating the "mental" disease-illness complex from the bodily disease-illness complex. Within the MMM-inclined theories things seem to become somewhat more complicated. While TMM-inclined theories focus on the "cause-side" of the disease-illness-health complex, and make 'disease' the basic concept, whereby the notion of illness therefore comes to play a secondary role, it is the other way around with the MMM-oriented theories. Since the focus is here on the "effect-side" of the disease-illness-health complex and 'health' (or 'ill-health') is made the basic concept, the notion of illness (which is the same as the notion of ill-health) becomes far more important to our discussion. Ill-health or illness is here not necessarily linked to disease. So we will have to face the possibility of a category of illness that is not due to disease. And since illness is characterized in terms of incapacitation on a whole-person level, it seems not to be evident how "mental illness" could be separated from bodily illness, or even whether such a distinction is necessary or desirable. This seems to be somewhat of an MMM-counterpart to the somaticist-TMM problems in separating bodily and "mental disease", though located at the "other end" of the disease-illness complex.

Keeping in mind that the Szaszian critique, after the disease-illness distinction has been taken into account, has been construed as primarily directed at the notion of mental *disease*, we should all the same take note of some difficulties that at least appear to attach to the MMM approach in this context. Suppose that we would want to retain the distinctions between "mental disease" and bodily disease and between "mental illness" and bodily illness. How would we arrive at this? We could either justify the disease-distinction in terms of the illness-distinction, and say that "mental" (as opposed to bodily) disease is disease that tends to produce "mental" (as opposed to bodily) illness. This would require that the "mental"-bodily illness distinction could be made without reference to the "mental"-bodily disease distinction. Or we could justify the "mental"-bodily illness distinction in terms of the "mental"-bodily disease distinction and say that "mental" (as opposed to bodily) illness is illness that is produced by "mental" (as opposed to bodily) disease. This would require that the "mental"-bodily disease distinction could be made without reference to the "mental"-bodily illness distinction. Now, since the kind of medical model under discussion here implies defining disease in terms of illness-producing tendencies, it would seem plausible to characterize "mental disease" as disease that tends to produce "mental illness" and bodily disease as disease that tends to produce bodily illness. This would however run into a number of counter-intuitive instances. A great variety of well-established physical diseases, particularly diseases of the brain and other parts of the central nervous system, produce effects on the "mental" part of the capacity-of-the-person level. These would then have to be re-classified as "mental diseases". The theories outlined previously, however, avoid this problem. They do this by, in a sense, giving up the "mental"-bodily illness distinction. Illness, in these theories, seems to be a neutral category, with regard to bodily and mental, in the sense that you could not without knowledge of the causes of a person's illness decide whether he was "mentally ill" or physically ill. So to retain the notions of "mental" and bodily illness, on this platform, it seems that you would have to rely on the second of the above-mentioned alternatives, viz. to justify the "mental"-bodily illness distinction in terms of the "mental"-bodily disease distinction. But this would not be sufficient. Because since illness on this view does not have disease as a necessary condition, we would have to take into consideration the possibility that the illness of a person is due to something other than disease. There seems to be a need of distinguishing illness-producing circumstances that are diseases from illness-producing circumstances that are not diseases.

One such distinction is made explicitly within the three theories. Diseases are distinguished from impairments and injuries, which are also types of illness-producing circumstances. This distinction is undoubtedly an important one from the point of view of clarifying medical concepts, but I think it is less important to our present purposes. I shall largely bypass this distinction. To avoid complicating our discussion I shall use "disease" in a broad sense, covering the class of "pathological" phenomena. This is in accord with Boorse's use of the term, which provides one more reason, if we want to avoid making comparisons too complicated, to disregard the distinction in our discussion. So the reader who might object to this simplification could substitute "disease or impairment or injury" for "disease" when used in the context of MMM-inclined reasoning in the following.

But let us before we press this point of the need of distinguishing among mental, incapacity-producing factors to arrive at a "mental disease" category try to get a clear view of the MMM-inclined approach. The focus, as mentioned, is on the whole-person-capacity level of analysis. A person is said to be in a state of health when his capacity to act satisfies certain criteria (somewhat differing among the three theories outlined) and ill when this capacity is compromised. Now of course a tremendous lot of widely different factors could impose restrictions on a person's capacities (ranging from poverty and snowstorms to religiously motivated self-mutilation). So a first delineation of illness-producing factors would have to be made by introducing the qualifier that incapacitations produced by internal factors are referred to when we speak of illness. This narrowing down of the illness-category is more or less explicitly made in the theories of Pörn, Whitbeck and Nordenfelt, which distinguishes them from some of the reasonings of opponents of Szasz whose views were discussed in chapter 3. So a first sub-categorizing of incapacitation-causing factors will be into the two categories of external and internal factors, where only the second is relevant to our discussion. But internal factors could also be of very diverse kinds. A first question to answer is if *all* instances of internally caused incapacitation are illness-instances according to these theories. And, as far as I can see, they are. We could then divide internal incapacity-producing factors into physical factors and mental factors. (Some would perhaps like to distinguish "spiritual" factors as a third sub-category, or a sub-sub-category among mental factors, but I shall, for the sake of simplicity, disregard this possibility.) And now we are beginning to approach the heart of the matter. Among the internal incapacity-producing factors a sub-class, that of diseases, should be delineated, and this class should be sub-divided into the class of bodily diseases and the class of "mental" diseases. These should show some common and some distinguishing characteristics.

What are the defining characteristics of disease in general, that "mental diseases" could be shown to embody? There seem to be, in general, two ways to arrive at these. The first way is to start from the "fact" that there are two sub-categories of phenomena called diseases, physical ones and "mental" ones, and go on to search for common characteristics of the two categories. Then you state that this set of common characteristics constitutes the defining characteristics of disease. The second way is to start from the assumption that physical disease is the basic and paradigmatic disease-type, and go on to search for the disease-defining characteristics among instances of physical disease. When these have been arrived at, you proceed to search for the presence (or non-presence) of the same characteristics among mental, illness-producing, phenomena.

We should note that the MMM-inclined theorists reviewed, at least Nordenfelt and Whitbeck, use the first approach. They actually build their concepts of mental disease into the general concept of disease right from the start. To Nordenfelt disease is a process internal to a person's body *or mind*, that tends to cause incapacitation.[11] And to Whitbeck disease is a *psycho*physiological process.[12] This implies having accepted the concept of mental disease at the onset of the analysis. Or, perhaps more correctly, it implies putting bodily and "mental" disease on a par with regard to how the characteristics of a general concept of disease should be described. This constitutes a disqualifying of my first methodological postulate, and should therefore not be accepted by me. From the premises of this study I would have to, when discussing on an MMM platform, just as I did when I discussed within the TMM framework, opt for giving preference to the second alternative above. That is, I should take 'physical disease' to be the more basic concept and proceed to investigate whether or not so-called mental disease is relevantly similar.

Generally speaking I believe there are two main approaches to showing that mental factors could be viewed as diseases analogous to bodily diseases. Either you could try to show, on theoretical grounds, that they satisfy exactly the same defining criteria that bodily diseases do (with regard to their status as disease.) Or you could opt for a quite different approach, and take full account of the value-dimension of the notion of disease, inherent in the MMM approach, and try to show that the sort of evaluations that pertain to the phenomena called mental diseases are completely analogous to bodily-disease evaluations. As for the second alternative, it is debatable whether the approach could be described as a fundamentalist one or not. This would depend on whether or not one claimed the evaluative dimension of disease-decisions to be a really distinguishing criterion, which would probably not be an easy route to take, or whether one opted for a somewhat more superficial pointing out of analogies between decisions regarding bodily and "mental" disease. I shall have something to say about both these possible approaches.

Now it should be kept in mind, just as was the case when we considered the TMM approach, that a basic feature of a medical model of abnormal behaviour and mental afflictions is that "mental diseases" should be shown to be on the one hand relevantly *similar* to bodily diseases in order to be reasonably included in the category of disesase in general, and on the other hand relevantly *dissimilar* to bodily diseases in order to justify the division of disease in general into two sub-classes. The first requirement entails showing that "mental disease" phenomena, through satisfying the criteria of disease in general, can be distinguished from phenomena that are not diseases. The second requirement entails showing that "mental diseases" satisfy some criteria that bodily diseases do not satisfy.

As for the second requirement, MMM-inclined theories seem to face no problems. The category of "mental diseases" is distinguished from the category of bodily diseases by way of the different internal factors (mental as opposed to bodily) that tend to produce illness. There appears to be no possibility of a somaticist position with the MMM approach. The only way to retain a somaticist view of "mental disease", within MMM-reasoning, would be to distinguish "mental" from bodily disease by way of pointing to a distinction between mental and bodily types of effects on the incapacitation-level. "Mental disease" would then be distinguished from bodily disease through its tendency to produce "mental" rather than bodily illness. The internal factors producing the "mental" illness could then well be physical. But illness (as well as its opposite, health) is, as we have noticed, a neutral category within this framework. A person's capacity or ability to act is a capacity of the person as a whole, not of his mental or bodily part. To speak of a person as "mentally" or physically ill (or healthy) would, it seems, require a justification in terms of the factors that produce his state of health or illness. And those could, of course, be bodily or mental. But then you could not divide the disease-types into mental and physical by way of pointing to the mental or bodily type of illness.

So "mental disease" would here have to be construed as genuine "mental disease" — that is, mental factors producing illness in a person. This would also entail, as far as I can see, that "mental diseases" believed to be, or proven to be, physically caused would have to be reclassified as physical diseases on the MMM platform. And the illness, should one want to keep the division into bodily and "mental" illness, of a person suffering from such a disease would have to be called a physical illness. This, it seems, might run into conflict with ordinary intuitions. Let us suppose that schizophrenia turned out to be physically caused, for instance by a genetic or bio-chemical abnormality. This would, with the MMM view, have to be spoken of as a physical disease, which seems quite appropriate. But the illness of the schizophrenia-afflicted person would also have to be spoken of as a physical illness, because the only plausible way of distinguishing bodily from "mental" illness, on the MMM platform, is by way of dividing the types of internal factors that cause the illness into physical and mental. This, however, might point more to ambiguities and complexities with regard to the uses of "disease" and "illness" and their relations in the area of the "mental" in general, than to problematic aspects of the MMM approach.

Now, with regard to the other requirement of a medical model of abnormal behaviour and mental afflictions, that of showing how to keep "mental disease" analogous to "bodily disease" and distinguished from non-disease, there might be more of a substantial problem with the MMM approach. Since illness with this approach could be due to other than disease-factors (non-illness is not the same as absence of disease, and disease and health, which is the same as non-illness, are not opposites), an important question is this one: How do we distinguish one sub-class, within the class of mental, illness-producing, factors, that satisfies the criteria of disease (the same disease-criteria, that is, that bodily diseases satisfy) and therefore constitutes the class of "mental diseases"? It seems that to be able to accomplish this we must use some criteria other than being mental, and illness-producing. One answer to this might be to deny that there are mental, illness-producing factors that are not "mental diseases". But this would run into a number of counter-intuitive examples. A person harbouring fanatically religious beliefs of a bizarre and irrational kind could be well imagined to suffer severe incapacitation as a consequence of those beliefs. A person in a state of grief would surely be incapacitated to some extent by this. (It should be noted, however, that among the MMM-inclined theorists reviewed, Nordenfelt has a special treatment of the condition of grief.[13]) A person being "madly" and unhappily in love with someone who did not return his feelings would be incapacitated by his emotional state. Yet we would hesitate to speak of any of those as "mentally diseased". All the same, they are all examples of persons afflicted by mental, incapacity-producing conditions.[14]

So, it seems, we would have to find a way of distinguishing among mental, illness- or incapacity-producing factors, thereby to enable us to tell which ones *are* "mental diseases" and which ones *are not*. Now, the way we ought to do this (according to postulate 1) would be by showing that "mental diseases" satisfy the criteria that make bodily diseases diseases, while non-"mental-disease"-type mental, illness-producing factors do not. Which are these criteria? The disease-definitions provided by Pörn, Whitbeck and Nordenfelt do not seem to assist us here in any self-evident way. We are told that diseases are processes that have a causal tendency to compromise health, health being in turn defined as capacity or ability to act in a certain desirable way.

One option now is to try to characterize "mental disease" in terms of dysfunction or of deviation from some normality of functioning, thereby attempting a distinction between mental, illness-producing factors that are normal in some sense, and mental, illness-producing factors that are abnormal in some sense. But would this not lead us into a characterization of "mental disease" in TMM-inclined terms? And would this not face the MMM approach with the same kind of difficulties that we discussed in the previous section? This depends on what kind of normality the "mentally diseased", as opposed to the non-diseased but equally mentally incapacitated, person is taken to deviate from. If we assume some kind of natural order of functioning as the standard of normality, we are faced with the same problem as the TMM theorist — that is, showing that there is a "natural order" of mental functioning in the same sense that there is one of physical functioning. And this difficulty, in the TMM case, consists largely, as we have seen, in establishing that standards of behaviour (through which mental functions could be inferred) and mental functions are not to some extent of a social and normative (as opposed to a biological/natural/descriptive) kind. But now it must be remembered that disease is not a value-free notion within MMM-reasoning. So perhaps the abnormality that would distinguish the "mental disease"-produced incapacitation from other kinds of mentally produced incapacitation *ought* to have a negative value attached to it in a way that is typical of "ordinary" disease but untypical of non-disease-type mental, incapacity-producing circumstances? This way the MMM approach would seem to escape some of the objections to, for instance, Boorse's attempt at establishing a reasonable concept of mental disease.

So what we would require here, from the protagonists of an MMM-inclined defence of the notion of mental disease, would be a demonstration of two matters: 1) that value-considerations in instances of the kind of abnormalities called mental diseases are analogous to value-considerations in typical cases of physical disease; and 2) that value-considerations in the "mental-disease" instances are disanalogous to value-considerations in instances of other mental incapacity-producing factors. If this could be accomplished the value-dimension of disease would serve as a criterion by which to delineate a "mental disease" category among internal, incapacity-producing circumstances.

I believe, however, that both these tasks could prove difficult to accomplish. Quite to the contrary, I think it could be shown that value-considerations in many instances of "mental disease" are not analogous to typical physical-disease evaluations, and that there is little difference between value-considerations of "mental disease" instances and evaluations of non-disease-type mental incapacity-producing circumstances.

The first of these two matters requires some elaboration. Let us assume that the value-component is one important component of diseasehood. That is, to say that something is a disease is to say (among other things) that it is something bad. So the first question is: Is the kind of badness that pertains to "mental disease" the same kind of badness that is implied in talking of physical disease, or is there some difference? On the face of it there might seem to be little difference. But, actually, some cases of "severe mental disease" would turn out to provide counter-instances to suggestions of analogous considerations.

Phenomena can be bad in various ways, or for various reasons. Criminal behaviour is said to be bad, because it constitutes the breaking of certain rules governing desirable and non-desirable behaviour. This is the kind of badness that calls for moral blame. Getting run over by a car is bad in another sense, primarily pointing to the fact that it hurts and incapacitates. Roughly the two kinds of "bad" could be distinguished along the lines: 1) bad on account of consequences for others than oneself, and 2) bad on account of consequences for oneself. To say that "mental disease" in a person is bad because it has non-desirable consequences for other people is putting it on a par with criminal behaviour. The claim that "mental disease", or "mentally diseased behaviour", is bad in this sense, would not in itself lead us to view it as analogous to physical disease. It would, on the contrary, direct us to point out a crucial difference between "mental disease" and physical disease, when it comes to the value-components of the two kinds of problems. A key problem in discussions of the value-status of "mental disease" seems to be that since assessments of "mental disease" must be built on assessments of behaviour, there is a strong tendency to arrive at mental-disease judgements via negative evaluations of behavioural abnormalities. And these seem often enough to be assessments of a bad-on-account-of-consequences-to-others kind. (Let us call this badness-type 1.) This is one reason why attempting to show that abnormal functioning in "mental disease" is analogous to abnormal functioning in physical disease is difficult, as we have seen in the previous section. But a medical model would not be applied to abnormal (in the alleged "mentally-diseased" sense) behaviour if this was all there was to it. The application of a medical model typically is tied to a bad-on-account-of-consequences-for-the-person-himself kind of negative evaluation. (Let us call this badness-type 2.)

The MMM approach implies regarding diseases as such on account of their tendency to produce states of incapacitation in a person, and it is strongly implicit that the badness of these incapacities is of the type-2 kind.

Now one problem with showing that evaluations of "mental" and physical disease are analogous is that badness-type 2 evaluations in many cases of "mental disease" must be performed by way of inference and hypothetical construction, in a way that need almost never be done in cases of physical disease. Many a person judged "mentally diseased" would flatly deny that his behaviour, or mental condition, is undesirable or bad from his own point of view. To account for the badness-type 2 ascription to the circumstances of such a person one has to revert to repudiating the person's ability to make such evaluations. Others will have to make them for him, or on his behalf. But this implies stating something like: "If this person were like the rest of us, then he would recognize that his behaviour or condition is undesirable or bad in the badness-type 2 sense." (Observe here that we are not now discussing the question of whether or not it is to be wished for, from some "objective" point of view, that the person should behave the way he does or harbour the mental conditions that he does. The question here is simply whether the value-component in "mental disease" is analogous to that pertaining to physical disease.) This seems rather unsatisfactory as a way of ascribing badness-type 2 to the "disease" of the person. How could such an ascription be validated? Let us suppose that the medical-psychiatric apparatus is put to work to change the person so that he actually becomes "like the rest of us" in various ways. Then we proceed to ask him: "Would you agree that your behaviour and mental condition, before the change were bad in the badness-type 2 sense?" If he does agree, would this be a validation of the correctness of the ascription of badness-type 2 to his behaviour and condition before the change? I think it would not. This would be no more of a validation than the opinion of any of "the rest of us" before the "change". His post-change agreement could well be interpreted as an expression of his value-system having changed as part of the overall change (which might, or might not, be a good thing; this is not the point). The fact remains that the badness-type 2 reasoning was not really applicable at the time when it was carried out. And therefore, it might be argued, "mental disease" evaluations of this type are not the same kind of evaluations as "ordinary disease" evaluations.

Let us now suppose that the person deemed "mentally diseased", after the medically-psychiatrically induced change has taken place, is asked the same question and answers in the negative. That is, he does not agree that his condition prior to the change was undesirable to himself. How would this be interpreted? Would it be conceded that the negative-value ascription before the change was wrongful? Or would we interpret his assessment of his behaviour and mental condition before the change as an indication that this person had not been thoroughly and successfully changed into one "like the rest of us" and that he therefore was not fit to judge the value-status of his former behaviour and condition? The first interpretation would entail concluding that this was an instance of "mental disease" where the value-status decision was disanalogous to the typical disease-value-status decision, which would point to a crucial difference between ordinary and (some cases of) "mental" disease. And this would pose a problem for those who argue that there are analogous value-elements in physical and "mental" disease decisions. The second interpretation (which I admit to believing the far more likely) would entail a number of intricate problems for the claiming of analogous value-decisions in "ordinary" disease and the discussed kind of "mental disease". It would appear that the criterion of a persons's fitness to judge on a matter of value, in this particular kind of disease, is a matter of his judgement being in conformity to the judgements of others. This sounds strange. It would also appear that a badness-type 2 evaluation here is something very different from what is the case in instances of ordinary disease. Here the badness-type 2 evaluation could not be contradicted, since the contradiction of it would imply unfitness to make such an evaluation. This in turn would imply that the use of badness-type 2 reasoning here is empty of all substance that would make possible an analogy with evaluations of ordinary disease. And a case could be made, I believe, for arguing that the kind of evaluation actually applied in these instances might upon closer analysis prove to come closer to a badness-type 1 evaluation. I shall not, however, pursue this line of thought in this context, since the primary object now was to discuss whether or not considerations concerning the value-status of disease could be in any evident way shown to be analogous in "ordinary" and "mental" disease.

But it could not be the case that all persons who, owing to some mental condition, refuse to acknowledge decisions regarding the undesirability of their state of capacity or incapacity, are disqualified from making such self-evaluations on account of the condition in question. A variety of mental "factors" or "conditions" could sustain a refusal to acknowledge other persons' negative evaluations of one's own state of capacity. The religious fanatic could again serve as an example. Such a person could, on account of his religiously motivated beliefs, systems of priorities etc., be in disagreement with others as to the evaluation of his present state of capacity, and this state of capacity could well be imagined to be severely compromised (from the majority point of view) by those very beliefs and priority-systems. But in this case we would not disqualify him from making his own assessments of the desirability or otherwise of his capacity-state. And we would certainly not suggest that the medical-psychiatric apparatus should be put to work on him to make him enough like "the rest of us" to change his notions of evaluation.

So to justify the difference in our views of the self-evaluative capacities of the religious fanatic and the "mentally diseased" person, we would, it seems, have to find some theoretical foundation providing non-evaluative criteria for our disqualifying of the "mentally diseased" person. And since the mental condition of the "mentally diseased" person that disqualifies him from making valid self-evaluations in fact is the same mental condition that produces the incapacities that we deem non-desirable — that is, the incapacities that serve as the distinguishing criteria of disease — this amounts to finding some theoretical grounds for the disease-status of the person.

So it seems that we are again directed to finding some non-evaluative way of establishing analogy between the "mental disease" type of phenomena and "ordinary" disease, preferably by pointing to some type of abnormality that could be characterized theoretically.

Now as regards the second of the two matters suggested on page 107 to be important — the one, that is, concerning the issue of using evaluative dimensions of the disease notion to delineate a category of mental disease among mental, incapacity-producing circumstances — it would appear that this could simply not be done with the aid of MMM theorizing. It seems that the negative value that pertains to disease is dependent on the fact that diseases tend to compromise something that has a positive value (health). But other mental factors (such as grief, being "unhappily in love", etc) *also* compromise a desirable state of capacity. On this point there seems to be no disanalogy of evaluation. The negative value that pertains to the effects on the capacity-level could not be used to distinguish between different categories of mental, incapacity-producing factors ("mental-disease" and non-"mental-disease" kinds, that is). It seems that what would be required to make the distinction between "mental diseases" and other mental, incapacity-producing circumstances (since we cannot here revert to claiming the former statistically abnormal or sub-par functioning as matched against a "species-design") is a way of judging the former as *in themselves* of negative value (normatively abnormal), *without* referring to their effects on the capacity level. And how this should be accomplished, on the MMM premises, I am unable to see.

Let us, finally, attempt yet another way to solve the dilemma of delineating a category of mental disease on the MMM approach. At this point I would like to, very briefly, bring into the discussion an aspect of the contribution of Peter Sedgwick.[15] Sedgwick has claimed vigorously that the attacks on the notion of mental disease that are based on the view that it is normative and evaluative, and the not very successful attempts to defend the same notion by trying to show that it is descriptive and non-evaluative, are equally flawed. The reason for this, Sedgwick claims, is that all notions of disease, mental and physical, are fundamentally evaluative and based on socially and culturally relative standards of what is desirable and what is not, as regards human bodily and mental functioning. There would simply not be any category of disease if we did not decide that certain phenomena are detrimental to certain human and social values. This very radically evaluative view of disease, which is as far as one can get towards the opposite of the Boorsian view on the question of the value-status of the disease-notion, immediately provokes the question whether *every* type of human abnormal functioning that has a negative value is a disease-instance. But Sedgwick answers in the negative, and it is his qualification of this answer that can be of interest for our present discussion. The way "mental" and bodily disease could be shown to be analogous, and at the same time be kept distinct from non-disease types of phenomena with a negative value-status is through being placed within a common structure of valuation *and* within a common structure of *explanation*. It is through placing "mental" as well as physical disease "within a relatively restricted set of causal factors operating within the boundaries of the individual human being",[16] that the disease-type of phenomena are distinguished from other forms of human functioning that have a negative value-status.

Could "mental disease" be claimed to be analogous to physical disease and disanalogous to other mental, incapacity-producing circumstances, on the MMM platform, by way of referring to a "common structure of explanation"? We would then require (according to postulate 1) that the structure of explanation of physical disease was first clarified, and then that it could be shown that the same structure of explanation was applicable to "mental disease" (but not to other mental, illness-producing factors). Now, without going into detail, physical diseases are typically explained in terms of diverse causal relations between changes of physical structures and subnormal functionings of physical systems. To show that "mental diseases" are explained analogously we could choose between 1) stating that "mental diseases" should also be explained in terms of physical structural and functional abnormalities, and 2) stating that there are mental structural and functional abnormalities very analogous to the physical ones. The first alternative is not open to the MMM approach for reasons given previously. The second alternative would require access to an encompassing theory of genuinely mental functionings. And now we seem to be back to the same problems that faced the TMM enterprise of establishing analogous disease-discourses in the physical and mental areas. We have to find a theory that is competent to provide a causal account of "mental disease". And we are equally back with the suspicion of metaphorical reasoning.

Psycho-analysis, suggested by Boorse to be the appropriate kind of theory to serve the purpose of establishing the relevant body function/mental function analogies, might perhaps satisfy MMM-inclined theorists as well. Let us assume that it does so satisfy them. Let us also assume, for the sake of discussion, that the psycho-analytic theoretical framework provides an explanatory account that is sufficiently like the explanatory account usually applied to physical-disease phenomena (this being, it should be noted, a rather controversial assumption) to make it plausible to speak of "a common structure of explanation". Will this explanatory structure provide us with grounds for distinguishing between "mental disease" phenomena and other mental, illness-producing phenomena? This is not evident. The psycho-analytic framework could of course give us a causal account of any mental, illness-producing circumstances that we would wish explained. It could explain in causal terms the conditions of grief, of being "unhappily in love", and of harbouring irrational and incapacitating religious beliefs, as well as the conditions called "mental diseases". This would not solve the dilemma before us.

But perhaps this is beside the point. Maybe we should interpret Sedgwick's suggestion in another way, viz. as meaning that diseases are distinguished from non-diseases (among functional deviations with a negative value-status) by being the type of phenomena that we *wish* to explain in terms of a certain structure of explanation (common to physical and "mental" disease). So the distinguishing feature of "mental diseases" (as compared with other mental, illness-producing conditions) would be that we tend to *want* to have them explained in causal (for instance psychoanalytical) terms, while we prefer to abstain from explaining other mental circumstances in such terms. This might well be so. But it would not bring us closer to solving our dilemma, since the question is precisely *why* we should view certain phenomena as "mental diseases" and therefore as preferably explainable within the framework of "the common explanatory structure of physical and 'mental' diseases", while other, equally incapacitating mental conditions should be kept out of this framework.

I believe we must, again, return to the notion of some abnormality, distinguishing "mental disease" type illness-producing factors from other mental, illness-producing factors. And this abnormality should not be expressed in terms of deviation from species-design, since this is not a disease-distinguishing criterion within MMM-inclined theorizing. And it could not be expressed in terms of its tendency to produce incapacitation on the whole-person level, since this would not exclude non-disease-type mental, illness-producing circumstances.

It seems to me that with regard to the MMM enterprise of establishing a reasonable notion of mental disease we here encounter a problem the path to whose solution is not immediately apparent.

What conclusions can we draw from the discussions of the MMM-approach to conceptualizing abnormal behaviour and mental afflictions in terms of disease? To make the MMM platform a powerful tool for rebutting the criticism of the concept of mental disease, it would, to begin with, have to be shown that it gives a characterization of the set of medical-model concepts which is superior to the characterization given by the TMM. Granted that this were so (which would of course be denied by adherents of a more Boorsian philosophy of health and disease), a number of objections could still be raised against the way "mental disease" is construed and delineated on this platform. The relations between "mental disease" and "mental illness" seem to prove more problematic with this approach than on the TMM platform. There seems to be an acceptance, on the part of the theorists reviewed, of the desirability of characterizing disease in general in a way that makes the notion of mental disease an integral part of the general concept from the start. This, I believe, is a consequence of accepting existing notions of health and disease as starting-points of the analysis, but it turns out to be hard to accept when we want to discuss critiques of existing notions. The major problem, however, I believe to be the difficulty in distinguishing the "mental disease" type of phenomena from other types of mental, illness-producing, phenomena. I would not claim that there is no way out of this dilemma. I would suggest, however, that the burden of taking the analysis further rests with the proponents of an MMM-inclined defence of the mental-disease concept. My aim has been, in accordance with the strategy of discussion chosen and outlined in chapter 1, to problematize this version of the medical-model conception; and, to the extent that my arguing has been reasonable, I believe that we have arrived at some substantial problems of the MMM approach.

Some concluding remarks

Let me try to summarize the outcome of the discussions undertaken in this chapter, and attempt some conclusions. Starting from the somewhat unsatisfactory results of the discussions of chapter 3, where the notions of a reasonable, up-to-date, medical model on the part of some of the opponents of Szasz, seemed to require further elaboration to become useful in a counter-critical strategy, I have in this chapter tried to help qualify those notions. Two ideal-type medical conceptual models, the TMM and the MMM, were sketched in chapter 4, each harbouring different basic assumptions as to the characterization of disease, illness and health. A number of up-to-date medical-philosophical theories were also outlined to substantiate the model-constructions. I then tried to problematize the possibilities of arriving at a reasonable mental-disease characterization on the platform of each one of the models. On page 79 I suggested that three issues seemed important in this problematization: the focussing on the "cause-side" (within TMM reasoning) or on the "effect-side" (within MMM reasoning) of the disease-illness-health complex; the viewing of disease as a value-free (within TMM discourse) or a value-laden (within MMM discourse) notion; and, to a lesser extent, the different ways of distinguishing disease from illness within the two models and the two groups of theories. My discussion has led me to the finding of problematic aspects of both models.

The TMM approach was suggested as including two differing strategies for defending a fundamentalist notion of mental disease: one based on a somaticist view, and the other based on a genuine-mental-disease view. By making bodily causes of "mental disease" problems a necessary condition of their disease status, the somaticist view seems to run the risk of making redundant the notion of mental disease. It seems difficult to make clear what is mental about "mental disease" if the pathology of it is a physical pathology. The genuine-mental-disease view, on the other hand, was found to face the problem of showing that the disease-characterization of physical disease is really applicable to so-called mental diseases. There is a problem in deciding what should be viewed as mental functions that are relevantly similar to bodily functional systems. And, given that such functional entities could be found, there remains the difficulty of showing that those could be said to fail to function in the same sense that a diseased bodily organ malfunctions. A well-established and valid theory of the mind would seem indispensable to such a demonstration. It is questionable whether psycho-analysis could provide the theoretical foundation that TMM-inclined defences of analogous reasoning on matters of physical and "mental" disease would need. A major problem with the TMM approach seems to be to establish that assessments of "mental disease" are value-neutral the way that physical-disease assessments (according to TMM spokesmen) are. Whether we speak of beliefs, desires, etc. as "functions", or we regard the psychoanalytic "Id", "Ego" and "Superego" as the proper mental functional "entities", it remains doubtful if evaluative standards of assessment could be kept out of our deeming them diseased. So, the TMM-inclined genuine-mental-disease attempt at constructing a reasonable mental-disease concept seems to fail primarily on the matter of showing that "mental diseases" are sufficiently similar to physical diseases.

The MMM, "effect-side-focused", platform for the defence of the mental-disease notion faces a somewhat different kind of problems. By making consequences on the whole-person-capacity level the defining characteristics of disease, this approach seems to run into difficulties in separating "mental diseases" from other mental, illness-producing, circumstances. At the root of this problem is the disease-illness relation that the MMM theorists reviewed claim to be the reasonable one. Since illness could here be due to something other than disease, it appears that the characterization of disease in terms of illness-producing circumstances is not sufficient to delineate a mental-disease category, unless we would want to expand this category to include a variety of mental, incapacity-producing circumstances that we do not ordinarily view as in any way pathological. The notion of a value-component of the disease-concept could not, according to our analysis, help solve this problem. The negative value-status of physical disease is not automatically applicable in many instances of so-called mental disease. The value-component of the disease notion could also not help us distinguish between "mental diseases" and other mental, incapacity-producing circumstances, because the negative value ascribed to disease seems to spring precisely from its illness-producing tendency. There is some reason to suspect that MMM-inclined reasoning, on the matter of delineating a "mental disease" category must at some point turn back to some sort of normality-abnormality distinction, and this would perhaps run into the same problematic need of solid and encompassing theorizing on matters of "the mental", that we saw TMM reasoning encounter.

On the issue of the disease-illness distinctions made within the two groups of theories, we found that the Boorsian way of viewing disease as a necessary condition of illness made the distinction quite unproblematic and irrelevant to the discussion of a reasonable notion of mental disease on the TMM platform. The disease-illness distinction made by Nordenfelt, Pörn and Whitbeck, on the other hand, appeared, when taken together with the necessity of construing mental disease as purely mental disease on the MMM platform, to entail some counter-intuitive consequences if one wants to retain the separation of "mental illness" from bodily illness.

The attempts at problematizing the possibilities of arriving at a reasonable and contradiction-free mental-disease notion on the TMM and MMM platforms, respectively, have been to some extent successful. Neither one of those platforms provides grounds for a self-evidently correct and reasonable conceptualization of abnormal behaviour and mental afflictions in terms of mental disease. I believe we are justified in remaining sceptical about the mental-disease notion, and in concluding that a theoretically motivated criticism of the medical-model conception of so-called mental-illness phenomena could not easily be refuted.

Notes

1 Boorse, C.: What a Theory of Mental Health Should Be.
2 Ibid. p. 66.
3 Ibid. p. 67.
4 Ibid.

5 de Sousa, R. B.: The Politics of Mental Illness, in *Inquiry*, 15, 1-2, 1977, pp. 187-202.

6 Ibid. p. 196.

7 Boorse, C.: What a Theory of Mental Health Should Be.

8 Ibid.

9 Ibid. p. 78.

10 One approach that could perhaps provide a basis for a more fruitful attempt to demonstrate analogies between bodily functional systems and mental functional systems is the computer-analogy approach to the theory of mind. (See, for instance, Boden, M. A.: *Minds and Mechanisms: Philosophical Psychology and Computional Models*, Brighton, Sussex, 1980.) It is far from self-evident, however, that this approach would provide grounds for a demonstration of analogous disease-status decisions in the areas of the physical and the mental, respectively.

11 Nordenfelt,L.: *On the Nature of Health*, p. 105.

12 Whitbeck, C.: A Theory of Health, p. 614.

13 Nordenfelt has a discussion concerning why, on his account, grief and other "negative" emotions are not diseases, though they are internal conditions that tend to produce incapacitation. The core of his argument is that the long-term minimal happiness of a person presupposes a variety and richness of his emotional life. This also includes a predisposition for negative emotions. (*On the Nature of Health*, pp. 114-116).

14 It should be noted that my argument here rests on the assumption that MMM-theorists find it urgent to avoid expanding the reference class of the term mental disease in a way that seems to come into conflict with ordinary usage. It is of course conceivable that they (or some of them) would instead accept such an expansion as a consequence of the disease definition they espouse.

15 Sedgwick, P.: Illness - Mental and Otherwise, in Caplan, A. L., Engelhardt, H. T., Jr. and McCartney, J. J. (eds.): *Concepts of Health and Disease*.

16 Ibid. p. 125.

6 "Mental illness", the medical model and ideology

Introductory notes

Chapters 2-5 have been aimed at testing the strength of a theoretically founded criticism, or questioning, of the medical-model conception of abnormal behaviour and mental afflictions through problematizing various efforts to defend that conception. If my reasoning has been fairly sound, we can conclude at least that the medical-model conception is not self-evidently unproblematic. The notion of mental disease seems to require further qualifying and defending, if we are to accept it as reasonably well-founded from a theoretical point of view. With this conclusion the major argument of this study is completed.

This final chapter will be devoted to briefly discussing some related issues, whose common denominator is that they involve foreseeable critical objections to strategical choices made in chapters 2-5. First I shall comment briefly on the choice of the notion of *mental disease* as the focus of attention in chapter 5, and discuss the option of retaining a reasonable notion of *mental illness* on the MMM premises as a partial rebuttal of the Szaszian type of critique. Second, I shall somewhat critically assess, and defend, the type of theoretical analysis adhered to in this study. And, third, I shall outline some steps to quite a different type of discussion of the medical-model conception of abnormal behaviour and mental afflictions: an ideological-critical one.

"Mental illness" and medical problems

I cannot tell to what extent the opponents of Szasz, discussed in chapter 3, would be happy with my efforts to help qualify and articulate their positions in chapters 4 and 5. It may well be that they would argue that the TMM-MMM distinction, and the theories of health and disease reviewed to substantiate that distinction, do not truly reflect *their* notions of what a medical model, that could plausibly apply to abnormal behaviour and mental afflictions, should look like. It is possible, for instance, that they would suggest that the focusing on the "effect-side" of the health-disease complex, that they seem to claim to be desirable, has not been carried out in a way that they would prefer. Should this be so, I frankly admit that I am at a loss to see what such a way might be. The theories reviewed to substantiate the TMM-MMM distinction are the most elaborate I have been able to find, and I find it hard to imagine some quite different theory, equally well systematized, that would escape the problematics arrived at.

But it could also be the case that the disease-illness distinctions prompted during the discussion by the theories reviewed, together with my subsequent stipulation of the notion of *mental disease* as the primary objective of the criticism — as well as of the defence — of the medical-model conception of so-called mental-illness phenomena, could be suggested to have blurred the issue. This might be a more substantial objection. Let us therefore try to get a somewhat clearer view of the significance of the various disease-illness distinctions with regard to the discussion of the medical-model conception of "mental illness" phenomena.

Let me recapitulate briefly the differing ways of distinguishing disease from illness that are employed by Boorse, on the one hand, and by Nordenfelt, Pörn and Whitbeck on the other. To Boorse illness is a subcategory of disease. All instances of illness *are* instances of disease, but not all instances of disease are instances of illness. To become an instance of illness an instance of disease must satisfy some additional criteria (besides the disease-criteria), primarily those of being incapacitating, of being undesirable to its bearer, of deserving treatment and of constituting grounds for excuse from moral blame. To Nordenfelt, Pörn and Whitbeck illness is a state of being incapacitated, that could, but need not, be a consequence or "effect" of the presence of a disease in the ill person. This leaves us with some interesting differences between the two approaches with regard to the discussion of the notions of mental disease and mental illness. The Boorsian theory, as it stands, obviously leaves room for the possibility that there could be "mental disease" without "mental illness". The MMM-inclined theories make possible the existence of "mental illness" that is not due to "mental disease". The strength of Boorse's approach, if it were to prove successful in establishing that purely mental conditions really could satisfy the TMM criteria of disease, would be that it would seem to escape some objections that are primarily directed at the notion of *mental illness* (on Boorse's version of illness). Much criticism of the notion of mental illness pertains precisely to the alleged unreasonableness of applying the criteria of being a title to special treatment and being a valid excuse for normally criticizable behaviour to this or that "mental illness" instance. If Boorse's theory were to ring true in its general characterization of disease and illness, that criticism might well be accurate in proving the notion of mental illness less valid, but it would not touch the notion of *mental disease*.

The MMM-inclined theorists, on the other hand, would, if their scheme of characterizing health, disease and illness in general were to prove superior, have proved that there is a plausible and accurate meaning of "mental illness" even if their approach should have proven less successful in establishing a plausible notion of mental disease. It is to this matter that I shall direct some attention. It is possible that some defenders of the notion of mental illness would be content with the plausibility of a notion of mental illness in a distinguished-from-mental-disease sense on the MMM premises, and view it as a partial rebuttal of the Szaszian type of critique. If my interpretation of this critique as primarily directed against the notion of *mental disease* is correct, this would, however, seem to be a mistake. "Mental illness", on the MMM premises, is, as we have seen, a category of human incapacitation that is not just devoid of any necessary relation to disease, but that furthermore would be seen to include a number of problematic human conditions that very few would regard as "mental illnesses" (in the undistinguished sense). It is hard to see how Szasz's criticism could be weakened by the acceptance of that mental-illness notion.

There is, however, yet another imaginable way of attempting a rebuttal of the Szaszian type of critique with the support of the plausibility of an MMM type of mental-illness notion (one, that is, that is not necessarily disease-related). An important aspect of the criticism from Szasz and others is the claim that so-called mental-illness phenomena are not, and should not be, properly viewed as *medical* problems. The major argument in favour of this claim is, of course, that "mental illness" phenomena, on Szasz's account, are not disease-type phenomena — and, Szasz would argue, medicine should stick to dealing with diseases. But maybe the latter suggestion is not self-evidently correct. There might be a case for viewing "mental illness" as a medical problem even if the notion of mental disease should be seen as untenable. This depends on what is a reasonable view of the relations between the notions of disease, illness and medical problem. Obviously an application of a medical conceptual model to certain abnormal behaviour and mental afflictions seems to entail stating that those problems are medical problems. And, equally obvious, the denial of the reasonableness of the application of the medical-model to the same phenomena seems to entail stating that they are not medical problems. Opponents as well as defenders of the application of the medical-model would certainly agree that there are problems that are not medical problems. So how would medical problems be distinguished from non-medical problems? We could distinguish two slightly, but importantly, differing ways to answer this question. We could state that medical problems are disease-type problems and nothing else. Or we could suggest that medical problems are problems that medicine as an art and science holds the legitimate expertise to deal with. One could argue that the two answers express the same idea if one espouses the notion that medicine holds the legitimate expertise to deal with diseases and nothing else. But one could also suggest that medicine holds the legitimate expertise to deal with diseases *and* with some other, non-disease-type, problems. It is the latter notion that is of some interest here. If medical problems are to be viewed as something more than disease-type problems, this would seem to open up a possibility for the problems called mental-illness problems being medical problems even if they are not disease-type problems. And if this is so, one dimension of the critique would seem misdirected. This would then constitute a sort of weakened form of defence of a medical-model conception of so-called mental-illness phenomena (as compared with the defence of their being mental-disease type phenomena discussed in chapter 5). The notion of medical problem would then work as a sort of bridging concept, through which it could be achieved that a "mental illness" problem would not have to be classified as a disease-type problem for it to be brought under medical jurisdiction.

Another way of stating the issue here is to say that what is at stake is psychiatry's status as a medical enterprise. A minimal requirement for such status would be that the problems that psychiatry deals with are medical problems. As we saw earlier, in chapter 4 pages 60, there are various, and quite contradictory, suggestions as to how psychiatry should react to the questionings of its status as a medical discipline. One strategy (exemplified by Ludwig[1]) is to narrow down the professed area of expertise of psychiatry to encompasse only such problems as are, or are believed to be, diseases in a very limited sense. Another (exemplified by Engel[2]) is to enlarge the scope of medical responsibilities, thereby ensuring that the type of phenomena that psychiatry deals with would seem properly medical problems. The latter strategy would seem in line with the matter we are here discussing — the one, that is, of trying to establish "mental illness" as a medical problem, even if it is not disease-related.

What is it that medicine deals with, typically, and that could be viewed as medical problems? We might recall Margolis' statement that "...medicine is an art of ministering to humans ...in terms of *pertinent* incapacitation...".[3] This seems to provide a wide enough characterization of medical activities not to risk drawing the line unduly narrowly around the area of medical problems. But the formulation also includes an important, and necessary, qualification. It expresses the notion that although medicine is an art of ministering to suffering and incapacitated humans, not every kind of human suffering and incapacitation is what medicine is an art of intervening against.

Obviously medicine deals primarily with diseases and disease-related human problems. But it is also true that medicine undertakes to assist people in solving problems that are not diseases. Problems in the context of childbirth are one example. Problems associated with the aesthetics of the human body (as in plastic surgery) are another. A third example is medical contributions to enhancing the performance of the human body (as in assisting athletes in their training). So, in one sense, it would perhaps be correct to say that medical problems include disease-problems and some other kinds of problems. But could this really provide grounds for viewing the "mental illness" type of problems (that are not caused by disease) as medical problems? Only in a very weak sense, I suggest. The obvious counter-argument would be that a case for regarding "mental illness" problems as medical problems, in a sense that would have *some* bearing on the Szaszian type of critique, should be built on a demonstration of similarities of those problems to the *core* of medical problems, not to fringe-type medical problems. It is by showing that "mental illness" shows affinities with the kind of problems that medicine could not shrink from taking responsibility for, that this weaker defence could gain credibility. And this would bring us back to a requirement of disease-status for the problems under discussion.

It should be noted that this attempt to view non-disease-related "mental illness" as a medical problem could find little support among the MMM-theorists themselves, that supplied the mental-illness notion that underpins the attempt. Whitbeck, especially, explicitly states that health-compromising conditions that are not diseases, injuries or impairments cannot reasonably be viewed as medical problems. She outlines a category of "self-alienating" conditions (including such problems as "motivational disturbances", "weakness of will", "self-deception" and "remorse/self-hatred") to substantiate this contention.[4]

I believe we must conclude that this weaker defence of the application of the medical-model to so-called mental-illness phenomena would have difficulty in achieving plausibility. If the MMM approach provides a reasonable characterization of illness, there might well be a plausible and accurate meaning to "mental illness", even if "mental disease" should prove to be a problematic notion. But this "mental illness" would on the first hand have very little to do with medical problems, and on the other be quite distant from the notion that was the target of Szasz's critique. The possibility of defending the medical-model conception of so-called mental-illness phenomena rests *either* on demonstrating that they are diseases, or disease-related, on theoretical grounds, *or* on showing that there are some other, extra-theoretical grounds for viewing them *as if* they were diseases. And the latter option brings us to some remarks on ideological dimensions of the mental-illness debate.

On ideological aspects of the medical-model conception of abnormal behaviour and mental afflictions

Some further remarks on the whys and hows of discussing the medical-model conception

In chapter 1, page 9, I suggested that there are mainly two ways to discuss the medical-model conception of abnormal behaviour and mental afflictions: one focusing on the theoretical or philosophical foundations of that conception, and one directed towards the ideological, social and political motives for, and functions of, that conception. I have chosen to keep the discussions of this study fairly well within the limits of the former way. The strategies adopted in the study could undoubtedly be challenged and criticized from several points of view. I shall comment on two foreseeable kinds of objections.

The line of argumentation pursued could perhaps be viewed as one of "fault-finding" and as one unduly inclined to problematizing; a purely deconstructive and "negativist" endeavour. My choice of platform, on the critical and "No"-answer side in the polemics over the reasonableness of the notion of mental illness or disease, has undoubtedly led me to direct my efforts towards actively searching out problematic aspects of various attempts to argue for a "Yes"-answer. Although I have certainly made an effort to find reasonable lines of defending the notion of mental disease or illness, this has been done with the purpose of questioning and problematizing them in the next step.

It is my contention that this mode of discussion can be defended and supported by a certain view of theoretical discussion in general. Such discussion, especially when it comes to arguing over issues that are controversial and where strongly opposing positions confront each other, should ideally proceed by argument and counter-argument. The aim of this study is to contribute to a, hopefully, continuing discussion about the theoretical underpinnings of the medical conceptualizing of abnormal behaviour and mental afflictions. I would not claim to have arrived at some final and irrevocable position. I would claim, however, that the burden of taking the argument in favour of the medical-model conception further rests with the proponents of that conception.

Quite a different kind of questioning of the strategy of discussion of this study, and one that could be raised by opponents as well as defenders of the notion of mental disease or illness, would be to state that the focusing on the theoretical or philosophical dimension of the polemics is a mistake. It is a bit naive, it could be argued, to believe that conceptual schemes, scientific and everyday, and their applications change and develop primarily on theoretical grounds. An analysis of the pros and cons of a certain conceptual apparatus, one could suggest, as well as an attempt to account for its scientific and everyday status, should be well anchored in an investigation into the social, political and ideological contexts in which it has grown and functions. Concepts of health, illness and disease, mental and otherwise, do not primarily gain status and become worked into our usage and reality-construction schemes on account of their theoretical coherence or logical consistency, and they are equally not abandoned on account of someone pointing out flaws in them in those respects. Thus might the argument go from the point of view of a pragmaticist defender of psychiatry, as well as from the point of view of an adherent of a critical sociology of knowledge.

I would agree with them to some substantial extent. It is quite possible that the decisive answers with regard to the issue of the feasibility of the medical-model conception of abnormal behaviour and mental afflictions should be sought for on levels of analysis other than theoretical. But, I would argue, this does not much diminish the value of theoretical discussion. It could not be denied that on one level of discussion there are *claims* made as to the medical-model of so-called mental-illness phenomena being theoretically well-founded, and *other claims* made as to the same model being theoretically invalid. Those claims would then preferably be discussed on the basis of thc *theoretical* arguments supporting them. And to deem the outcome of such a discussion irrelevant to what should count as a reasonable position on the appropriateness of a notion of mental disease or illness would seem dubious.

Quite another thing is that a discussion of the theoretical dimensions of the issue of the mental-disease notion would need supplementing with a discussion of extra-theoretical, and perhaps most importantly ideological, aspects of it. I shall devote the remainder of this chapter to some remarks on ideological dimensions of the medical-model conception of so-called mental-illness phenomena. A full-blown ideological-critical discussion would require a study of its own. I shall limit my remarks to suggesting some possible aspects of such a discussion.

Mental disease as a metaphor

We shall now leave the part of the discussion that is built on the TMM-MMM distinction, and return to a more general level of discussion, equivalent to the one in chapters 1-3, of the mental-illness notion. We shall thereby also for the remainder of the chapter drop the disease-illness distinction. "Illness" and "disease" will in the following be used as synonyms.[5]

In chapter 4, page 64, I distinguished between two ways to argue in favour of the appropriateness of using the term "mental illness": a fundamentalist and a metaphorist way. The fundamentalist approach implies arguing that "mental illnesses" or "diseases" are illnesses or diseases in exactly the same sense as physical illnesses or diseases — that is, it implies arguing that "mental illness" or "disease" satisfies the criteria of illness or disease in general. The metaphorist approach implies arguing that there are some good reasons for proposing that "mental illnesses" or "diseases" should be viewed *as if* they were diseases. Chapter 5 was devoted to discussing various attempts at defending the fundamentalist approach.

In my first postulate (page 11) I stated that the feasibility of applying a concept of mental illness to so-called mental-illness phenomena should be argued for by way of demonstrating that these phenomena are relevantly similar to "ordinary" or physical illnesses. As regards "relevantly similar", in chapter 5, when the fundamentalist argument in favour of the mental-disease notion was discussed, I have taken this to mean "similar in the sense of satisfying the same criteria of disease-status". The comparison-postulate should, I suggest, be applied also in a discussion of the pros and cons of a metaphorist argument. That is, if it is to be proposed that so-called mental-illness phenomena should be viewed *as if* they were diseases, the justification for this proposal would have to take the form of pointing to some characteristics that are shared by those metaphorical diseases and genuine diseases (even if it should be admitted that the metaphorical diseases did not share the defining characteristics of genuine diseases). Of course there are a number of dimensions along which so-called mental-illness phenomena could be compared to physical diseases. The question of the appropriateness of a metaphorist notion of mental illness or disease would reasonably revolve around the issues of, first, *which* dimensions of comparison should be deemed relevant, and, second, whether or not so-called mental-illness phenomena really *are* similar to physical diseases along those dimensions. I suggest that those dimensions would primarily be of a social or ideological nature in a wide sense. Before turning to a suggested scheme of discussing those dimensions of comparison, some remarks on the notion of metaphor should be made.

I shall follow Turbayne[6] in outlining the characteristics of a metaphor. To speak of something metaphorically is to speak of this something as if it was something else. Turbayne calls this "sort-crossing".[7] But it must also be the case that we are aware that the something we speak of is not really what we say it is. When we say, with Seneca, that man is a wolf, we do not actually mean that man is a wolf; we make believe that he is. But again, this make-believe is not totally without grounds (as viewed by the metaphor user). Turbayne expresses this as "I do not merely pretend that man shares the properties of wolves; I intend it."[8] That is to say that the wolf-metaphor of man implies that man shares some of the characteristics of wolves, and the use of the metaphor is intended to highlight precisely those characteristics in man. We use the term wolf in two senses and make believe that we use it in only one sense. Metaphors are often used to produce shifts in attitudes. By stressing some aspects of a phenomenon and suppressing others, a metaphor is a powerful tool in making and remaking our ways of viewing and evaluating the phenomenon in question. And as long as we are aware of the metaphorical status of a certain way of referring to a phenomenon, the use of a metaphor cannot be spoken of as a mistake. It can always, however, be assessed in terms of appropriateness and plausibility. A mistake, on the other hand, writes Turbayne, occurs when we lose sight of the metaphorical status of a word or designation. If we drop the "as-if" character of a certain way of speaking of a phenomenon, we are not merely re-allocating attitudes, but re-allocating facts. This, in Turbayne's vocabulary, is not only "sort-crossing", but "sort-trespassing".[9] If we take a metaphorical sense for a literal sense, we are not using a metaphor, but being used by it, writes Turbayne.

Metaphors have a common history of development. The introductory phase of a metaphor is characterized by the use of a word being simply inappropriate. To give a phenomenon a name belonging to something else is breaking a convention. This will in most cases evoke protest and denial, "since 'x' is not really a 'y'". But if the metaphor is an effective one this denial of its literal truth will serve to establish the dual meaning of the word in question. There will be a literal and a metaphorical sense in calling something a "y". This means that the metaphor is accepted precisely as a metaphor; we take part in the make-believe. During this, the second stage of a metaphor, it is used with an awareness of its metaphorical status. But in some cases the metaphor will tend to lose its metaphor-character — or, more correctly, it will cease being used as a metaphor. The make-believe sense in which it is used will tend to grow weaker, and eventually disappear. To use the word will now mean to speak literally of something. This means that special sets of implications have, by this stage, been invented for the "y", designated to explain facts about the "x's". The "x's" are now literally a special kind of "y's". "The long continued association of two ideas, especially if the association has theoretical and practical benefit, tends to result in confusing them",[10] writes Turbayne. This confusion is aided by several factors. To begin with, it is of importance that the two ideas actually have their name in common. This circumstance in itself tends to facilitate the belief in identity. "Second, we are not always told that the two ideas are really different...Third, even when we are told, we export properties from one idea to another, such being the nature of metaphor."[11] All this amounts to the possibility that a metaphor may become so well established in a certain way of construing reality, and speaking about it, that virtually no one recognizes its metaphor status. Then we are "victims" of the metaphor in the sense that it really governs our ways of construing reality.

So much for reviewing Turbayne on metaphors. Now this account of why and how a metaphor could be used certainly could apply to the term "mental illness" or "mental disease". This might appeal to defenders as well as to critics of the notion of mental illness. Thomas Szasz, as we saw, tends to view "mental illness" this way. Another critic of the mental-illness notion, Theodore Sarbin,[12] has made an ambitious attempt to demonstrate that the term "mental illness" came to be applied to abnormal behaviour and mental afflictions for quite non-theoretical reasons. The metaphorical status of the term was, according to him, quite openly stated in the beginning, and the "make-believe" consisted in viewing minds as entities that really could be ill or diseased in the same sense that bodies could. The motives, he suggests, were originally humanitarian, and the aim was to rescue individuals from the claws of the witch-hunting inquisition. But gradually, writes Sarbin, the "as-if" was dropped, and the metaphor was reified into a term with a nowadays allegedly literal meaning, that there seems almost no hope of doing away with.

I shall make no attempt, in this context, to assess the reasonableness of viewing "mental illness" as a third-stage metaphor. This would require an in-depth investigation into the history of the notions of mind and mental illness. For my present purpose, which is to establish some grounds for a tentative sketch of an ideological-critical discussion of the medical-model conception of so-called mental-illness phenomena, it is sufficient to highlight some features of the nature of metaphor. I believe a distinction can be made between two main purposes of using a metaphor. One is to use it because one believes that this would contribute to the *understanding* of some phenomenon. The other is to express an *evaluation* of a phenomenon. An example of the former is the machine-metaphor of the human body. Although calling the human body a machine, in most cases, would not imply claiming that it is a machine, it would imply claiming that the machine view of the human body facilitates understanding some features of the workings of it. An example of the second use of metaphor is calling the abuse of narcotics a "cancer in the body of society". Although this might also have some purpose related to understanding or explanation, the main purpose is probably to express an evaluation of narcotics-abuse as dangerous, horrifying and urgently to be avoided, from a societal point of view. The shift of attitudes towards a phenomenon, that can be accomplished by a powerful metaphor, as described by Turbayne, is probably most effective on an emotional level of operation.

Another basic feature of metaphor is that it is not a mistake to speak metaphorically of something. The application of a metaphor to a phenomenon is perfectly legitimate, as long as the metaphor-status remains in the open. Since the phenomenon to which the metaphor is applied does not share all, or even the most central and defining, characteristics of the phenomenon from which the designation is borrowed, the application of the metaphor could always be challenged from the point of view of appropriateness. Since the metaphor stresses some features of the phenomenon to which it is applied, and disregards others, the important questions to ask would be what good reasons there are for highlighting precisely those aspects of the phenomenon in question, and what consequences this highlighting has. A metaphorist defence of the conceptualization of certain abnormal behaviours and mental afflictions in terms of "mental disease", would then preferably consist in arguing for the feasibility of stressing some, disease-analogous, aspects of those behaviours and afflictions, and for the positive consequences of this stressing. A criticism of the metaphorist approach would consist in demonstrating primarily that there are good reasons for not stressing those very aspects, and/or that other aspects should be stressed, for some reason, and/or that the consequences of stressing the aspects in question are other than was intended.

But in a discussion of what is to be wished for when it comes to highlighting certain aspects of so-called mental-illness phenomena and disregarding others, and when it comes to what should count as good or bad consequences, a number of questions quickly surface, of the following type: "To be wished for from what point of view?". "Good consequences according to whose assessment?" etc. The possibility of differing and conflicting interests, and of diverging assessments of the appropriateness of the metaphor of mental illness, becomes imminent as soon as we stop relying on a fundamentalist argument (stating that so-called mental illnesses or diseases are diseases, whether you like it or not). And this is exactly why the metaphorist approach should be discussed primarily within the context of an ideological-critical approach.

Ideological functions of conceptual models

It is a commonplace within several traditions of the sociology of knowledge and within many theories of ideology that conceptual models do not serve only (or, some would add, even primarily) theoretical purposes. Schemes of conceptualizing some part of reality grow and develop and change in a social context where scientific interests co-exist with, and intermingle with, social, political, economic and other extra-scientific forces in a way that makes the understanding and evaluation of the nature of a certain way of construing and comprehending some part of reality a matter of complex social analysis. Ideological functions of the application of a conceptual model to a certain area of problems or phenomena are perhaps among the most important to analyze in a discussion of the status, legitimacy and appropriateness of the model in question.

What is to be meant, more specifically, by "ideological functions"? The notion of ideology is a complex and multifaceted one.[13] It would hardly serve our purposes, in this brief outline of some starting-points of an ideological-critical discussion, to go into a detailed examination of various ways of explicating and using it. I shall stipulate roughly what I shall take to be the meaning of "ideology", and I suggest that this characterization comes close to the core meaning of "ideology" in many (though perhaps not all) current usages. Ideology designates a certain view, or interpretation, of certain phenomena that is associated with, and serves, certain specifiable interests. Those interests could be those of a smaller or larger group of people (for instance a social class or a profession) or of a society or a culture as a whole. The ideological function of a conceptual model would then consist in its application to certain phenomena having the result that those phenomena were viewed or interpreted or categorized in a way that served certain interests (and perhaps thereby disrupted certain other interests).

Now it should be noted that a discussion of the medical-model conception of abnormal behaviour and mental afflictions from ideological points of view has a significance of its own, regardless of whether a metaphorist or a fundamentalist approach underpins it. Critics of that conception sometimes construct their argument along the lines that *since* there seems to be a shaky theoretical foundation of the medical-model conception of so-called mental-illness phenomena, it becomes important to discuss the social and ideological functions of that conception. But of course this ideologically oriented discussion is, in a sense, interesting and important *regardless* of the strength of the theoretical defence of that conception. Even if the medical-model conception of so-called mental-illness phenomena could be shown to be theoretically well-argued there might be a case for criticizing its social and ideological implications. And, vice versa, if the theoretical foundation of this conception were unequivocally shown to be shaky, there might be convincing ideological motives for retaining it all the same. So, in one sense, the ideologically oriented discussion could be seen as independent of the more theoretical deliberations. But, of course, the importance of the outcome of a discussion of the ideological dimension would seem to grow in reverse proportion to the strength of the theoretical argument in favour of the medical-model conception. And from the point of view of a purely metaphorist defence of that conception, the outcome of an inquiry into the ideological functions of it would seem decisive with regard to its reasonableness or otherwise.

Steps to an ideological-critical discussion of the medical-model conception

In the following I shall briefly sketch some strategies for an ideological-critical discussion of the medical-model conception of so-called mental-illness phenomena and point out tentatively some directions in which such an analysis would take us.

One way to get a clear view of the ideological dimensions of the medical-model conception would be to confront, and contrast, it with a very different, non-medical, model of the same phenomena. I suggested in chapter 1 that major parts of the debate on psychiatry could be characterized in terms of a clash between two perspectives: a medical-humanitarian one and a sociological-critical one. Associated with the sociological-critical perspective is the application of a sociological conceptual model, which I suggest to be the most radically non-medical alternative conceptual scheme. The key feature of that model is the characterization and classification of so-called mental-illness phenomena as a sub-class of *social deviance*. This model could be specified along somewhat different lines. Just to give some substance to the notion of a sociological, non-medical, conceptual scheme of so-called mental-illness phenomena, I shall briefly outline the features of one version of it. Thomas J Scheff[14] has utilized a purely sociological conceptual apparatus to structure his labelling-theory approach to the problems of "mental illness". The kernel notion of his approach is that so-called mental-illness phenomena are preferably characterized as a sub-category within the category of social deviance. The behavioural deviances that tend to be labelled "mental illnesses" make up a residual category of rule-breaking behaviours alongside, and analyzable on a par with, other more established and more clearly specifiable categories, such as criminal behaviour, drug abuse, prostitution, etc. The theory is developed in explicit opposition to the medical view of "mental illness", and it is strongly suggested that a social systems model (as opposed to the individual systems models of psychiatry and psychology) is superior in characterizing (as well as explaining) on the one hand the social processes of "mental illness" ascription and societal intervention against "mental illness" phenomena, and on the other hand the communicative, interactional and experiential problems of the "mentally ill" themselves (that are not really "ill" or "diseased" at all on Scheff's terms). I shall in this context disregard the various problematic aspects of Scheff's theory, as a theory (concerning among other things its empirical status, its explanatory value and its internal coherence), and concentrate solely on the conceptual model around which it is built.[15] And this model, it should be repeated, puts "mental illness" phenomena on a par with other kinds of socially deviant behaviour when it comes to their primary characteristics.

We would thus start our ideological-dimension discussion with two opposing conceptual models, each claiming to provide a reasonable characterization of so-called mental-illness phenomena, one putting them on a par with "ordinary", or physical, diseases and one suggesting them to be on a par with social deviance, like criminal behaviour.

Now, if we accept the notion that conceptual models (especially if their key notions are to be viewed as metaphors) serve, or are supposed to serve, ideological purposes, the confrontation of the two models would facilitate highlighting the ideological aspects. The two models, through characterizing so-called mental-illness phenomena in very different ways, will work as ideological tools, by shifting our attention to different aspects of the "mental illness" complex. Each model will highlight some aspects and directly or indirectly obscure other aspects. You could view them as ideological filtering-screens, that tend to steer our perception of the "mental illness" problems in diverging directions. And this highlighting and obscuring will tend to affect our interpretative inclinations as well as our attitudes.

From the point of view of defending a metaphorist argument in favour of applying a medical model to so-called mental-illness phenomena, the ideological implications of that application would be seen as beneficial to the "mentally ill" themselves. By stressing and highlighting the similarities to "ordinary", or physical, disease the medical model will make us primarily view the "mentally ill" person as a suffering and incapacitated individual. The categorization of his problems as disease will be seen as a humanitarian effort to achieve social-role adjustments that are in the person's own interest. By granting him entrance to the social role of the diseased person a number of socially significant consequences, purportedly of value to him, will come into being. Perhaps most important is the removal of moral responsibility from the person with regard to his behaviour and condition, and his entitlement to help and support for relieving him of his problem. With the diseased-status would come also a benevolent and sympathetic attitude on the part of society and a lessening of demands and expectations of performance in various dimensions of social life. With this stressing of similarities of so-called mental-illness phenomena to "ordinary", or physical, diseases follows also a characterization of the interventions and practices aimed at solving the problems in question. These efforts will, in accordance with the medical ethos, be seen as a humanitarian attempt to alleviate the suffering and reduce the incapacitation of the person categorized as suffering from "mental illness". The purpose of these actions will be seen as self-evidently in accordance with the interests of the "mentally ill" person, even in those cases when he might not realize this himself.

Viewed through the filtering-screen of the sociological conceptual model, matters will seem quite different. Through focusing on those parts of the "mental illness" complex that share some characteristics with social deviance in general (and filtering out other parts), the sociological conceptual model makes us see an infringer of social norms rather than a suffering individual in the person labelled "mentally ill". The changes in the social status of the "mentally ill" person will be questioned from the point of view of whose interest they are really serving. The degrading and pejorative elements that the social status of "mentally ill" (as opposed to the social status of physically ill) carries will be highlighted, and the positive value of liberation from moral guilt (as viewed through the medical-model scheme) will be contrasted with the negative and dehumanizing effects of removal of moral responsibility and accountability. Where the medical-model screen made us see entitlement to treatment, the sociological model will make us see primarily obligations to change and adapt. And the interventions and practices directed against "mental illness" problems will be seen as social-control measures, aimed at converting an infringer of social norms into a social conformist. The primary interests that those interventions serve will, with this model, tend to be viewed as those of society at large, or of those who stand to gain from the retention of status quo of the social norm system.

This sketchy, and perhaps a bit over-dramatized, outline of the importance of the divergence of the foci of the two conceptual models should suffice to make clear the possibilities of pursuing an ideological-critical discussion along the lines of confronting and contrasting the two models. Obviously a number of aspects would have to be substantially articulated and elaborated in a full-blown analysis of ideological implications, motives and functions. Some necessary distinctions should be made, to serve as parts of the analytical structure of the discussion. I suggest the following distinctions to be of primary importance of a fruitful analysis. First, ideological *motives* should be distinguished from ideological *functions*. These need not coincide. The motives for applying a medical-model view to abnormal behaviour and mental afflictions might be supported by ideological inclinations that differ more or less from the ideological functions that this view actually comes to fulfil.

Second (and this has some bearing on the first distinction), different *levels of analysis* should be distinguished, and what is most important is probably to keep distinct an *individual* level and a *societal* level. Already the above sketch indicates that the medical-model "filter" tends to have an individual-level orientation, while the sociological model tends to turn our attention to societal-level considerations.

And, third, we should distinguish between *intra*-ideological and *inter*-ideological analyses. The former would consist in turning critical attention to psychiatric theorizing and practice on the basis of the very ideological premises that are (or are assumed to be) supported by a large consensus in our society and that supposedly underpin the activities of our societal-institutional agencies. The inter-ideological kind of critique would consist in investigating the accepted and promoted ideological premises themselves, and the role of psychiatry in enhancing and perpetuating them, from some ideological platform of a more "utopian" nature.

A necessary step in this analysis would undoubtedly also be to sub-categorize among so-called mental-illness phenomena. The class of phenomena to which the term "mental illness" might be taken to refer is certainly a very heterogeneous one, and the characteristics of showing affinities to "ordinary" disease and "ordinary" social deviance, respectively, might be very unevenly distributed among members of that class. The same heterogeneity would apply to psychiatric activities and interventions, which should also be taken into account.

I do not claim that this suggestion of the hows of an ideological-dimension discussion regarding the medical-model conception of so-called mental-illness phenomena is very original. As I have stated several times in this study, many critics of that conception have, explicitly or implicitly, founded their criticism on the adoption of a sociological-critical perspective and a sociological conception of the phenomena in question. What I suggest, however, is that an ideological-dimension analysis should be performed from a rather more neutral platform. The two models — the medical or illness model and the sociological or deviance model — should both be critically analyzed with regard to the outcome of their applications to so-called mental-illness phenomena. Various concrete cases of "mental illness", as well as of psychiatric activities, should be scrutinized from the point of view of the diverging ways the filtering screens of the two conceptual models respectively would make us conceive of them. And the diverse interpretations and evaluations the models would make us inclined to make, in substantial case by case comparisons, should be separately weighed and tested for reasonableness. The analysis should ideally be performed with a mind open for the possibility that both models provide opportunities to see clearly things that ought to be seen, and that the opposing model would tend to make us filter out.

I would not venture to suggest the likely outcome of a thorough ideological-critical analysis along the lines here suggested. I am inclined to believe, however, that it would produce arguments for, *as well as* against, a metaphorist defence of the medical-model conception of abnormal behaviour and mental afflictions.

Notes

1 Ludwig, A. M.: The Psychiatrist as Physician.
2 Engel, G. L.: The Need for a New Medical Model.
3 Margolis, J.: The Concept of Mental Illness: A Philosophical Examination, p. 7.
4 Whitbeck, C.: A Theory of Health, pp. 521-523.
5 This returning to the synonym use of "illness" and "disease" is motivated partly by a wish to simplify matters of expression and partly by the fact that some writers referred to in the following adopt the interchangeable use of these terms.
6 Turbayne, C. M.: *The Myth of Metaphor*, New Haven, 1962.
7 Ibid. p. 11.
8 Ibid. p. 15.
9 Ibid. p. 22.
10 Ibid. p. 26.
11 Ibid. p. 26.
12 Sarbin, T. R.: The Scientific Status of the Mental Illness Metaphor, in Plog, S. C. and Edgerton, R. B. (eds.): *Changing Perspectives in Mental Illness*, New York, 1969.

13 A good introduction to the problematics of the concept of ideology and an overview of various theories of ideology is provided by Larrain, J.: *The Concept of Ideology*, London, 1979.

14 Scheff, T. J.: *Being Mentally Ill*: A Sociological Theory, Chicago, 1966.

15 Thomas Scheff's labelling theory approach was an influential contribution to the intense debate on "mental illness" of the late 1960's and the 1970's. In contemporary sociological discussion it is often argued that labelling theory has lost much of its importance, as a general sociological approach to social deviance as well as when it comes specifically to its application to "mental illness" problems. I believe this dismissal of the approach to be premature *particularly* from the point of view of the need of a vitalized discussion of basic issues in the "mental illness" field. I suggest that the labelling theory approach — through the very radically sociological conceptual model it utilizes — still provides one of the more fruitful and interesting *sociological* perspectives on "mental illness" and I have tried to substantiate and elaborate that suggestion in Svensson, T: *Residual Deviance, Insanity Ascription and Social Order,* Studies on Health and Society no. 22, Department of Health and Society, Linköping University, 1994.

Bibliography

Ackerknecht, E. H. (1968), *A Short History of Medicine*, New York.

Ausubel, D.P.(1967), Personality Disorder Is Disease, in Scheff, T. (ed.): *Mental Illness and Social Processes*. New York.

Boden, M. A. (1980), *Minds and Mechanisms: Philosophical Psychology and Computational Models*, Brighton, Sussex.

Boorse, C. (1976), What a Theory of Mental Health Should Be, in *Journal for the Theory of Social Behaviour*, 6, pp. 61-84.

Boorse, C. (1977), Health as a Theoretical Concept, in *Philosophy of Science*, 44, pp. 542-573.

Boorse, C. (1981), On the Distinction between Disease and Illness, in Caplan, A. L., Engelhardt, H. T., Jr. and McCartney, J. J. (eds.): *Concepts of Health and Disease*, Reading, Massachusetts.

Brody, B. (1981), Szasz on Mental Illness, in Caplan, A. L., Engelhardt, H. T., Jr. and McCartney, J. J. (eds.): *Concepts of Health and Disease*, Reading, Massachusetts.

Brody, B. A. and Engelhardt, H. T., Jr. (eds.) (1980), *Mental Illness: Law and Public Policy*, Dordrecht.

Caplan, A. L., Engelhardt, H. T., Jr. and McCartney, J.J. (eds.) (1981), *Concepts of Health and Disease*, Reading, Massachusetts.

Conrad, P. and Schneider, J. W. (1980), *The Medicalization of Deviance*, St. Louis.

Engel, G. L. (1981), The Need for a New Medical Model, in Caplan, A. L., Engelhardt, H. T., Jr. and McCartney, J. J. (eds.): *Concepts of Health and Disease*, Reading, Massachusetts.

Feinstein, A. (1967), *Clinical Judgement*, Baltimore.

Flew, A. (1975), *Crime or Disease*, London.

Fitzpatrick, R. M. (1982), Social Concepts of Illness and Disease, in Patrick, D. L. and Scambler, G. (eds.): *Sociology as Applied to Medicine*, London.

Foucault, M. (1976), *Madness and Civilization - A History of Insanity in the Age of Reason*, London.

Langer, S. K. (1976), *Philosophy in a New Key*, Cambridge, Massachusetts.

Larrain, J. (1979), *The Concept of Ideology*, London.

Leifer, R. (1969), *In the Name of Mental Health. The Social Functions of Psychiatry*, New York.

Ludwig, A. M. (1975), The Psychiatrist as Physician, in *Journal of the American Medical Association*, 234, 6, pp. 603-604.

Macklin, R. (1981), Mental Health and Mental Illness: Some Problems of Definition and Concept Formation, in Caplan, A. L., Engelhardt, H. T., Jr. and McCartney, J. J. (eds.): *Concepts of Health and Disease*, Reading, Massachusetts.

Margolis, J. (1980), The Concept of Mental Illness: A Philosophical Examination, in Brody, B. A., and Engelhardt, H. T., Jr. (eds.): *Mental Illness: Law and Public Policy*, Dordrecht.

Miller, P. (1986), Critiques of Psychiatry and Critical Sociologies of Madness, in Miller, P. and Rose, N. (eds.): *The Power of Psychiatry*, Cambridge.

Moore, M. S. (1983), Some Myths about "Mental Illness", in Vatz, R. E. and Weinberg, L. S. (eds.): *Thomas Szasz: Primary Values and Major Contentions*, New York.

Nordenfelt, L. (1987), *On the Nature of Health. An Action-Theoretic Approach*, Dordrecht.

Nordenfelt, L. and Lindahl, B. I. B. (eds.) (1984), *Health, Disease and Causal Explanation in Medicine*, Dordrecht.

O'Connell, R. A. (1988), Psychiatry and Antipsychiatry, (a review of Roth, M. and Kroll, J.: The Reality of Mental Illness), in *American Journal of Psychiatry*, 145, 8, p. 1025.

Oxford Advanced Learner's Dictionary of Current English, (A.S. Hornby, ed.) (1987), eighth impression, Oxford.

Pies, R. (1983), On Myths and Countermyths, in Vatz, R. E. and Weinberg, L. S. (eds.): *Thomas Szasz: Primary Values and Major Contentions*, New York.

Plog, S.C. and Edgerton, R.B. (eds.) (1969), *Changing Perspectives in Mental Illness*, New York.

Pörn, I. (1984), An Equilibrium Model of Health, in Nordenfelt, L. and Lindahl, B. I. B. (eds.): *Health, Disease and Causal Explanation in Medicine*, Dordrecht.

Reading, A. (1979), Illness and Disease, in *Medical Clinics of North America*, 61, 4, pp. 703-710.

Redlich, F. C. and Freedman, D. X. (1986), *The Theory and Practice of Psychiatry*, New York.

Ross, A. (1979), Sygdomsbegrebet, in *Bibliotek for laeger*, 171, 2, pp. 111-129.

Ross, A. (1979), Opgør med antipsykiatrien, in *Bibliotek for laeger*, 171, 4, pp. 241-267.

Roth, M. (1976), Schizophrenia and the Theories of Thomas Szasz, in *British Journal of Psychiatry*, 129, pp. 317-326.

Roth, M. and Kroll, J. (1986), *The Reality of Mental Illness*, Cambridge.

Sarbin, T. R. (1969), The Scientific Status of the Mental Illness Metaphor, in Plog, S. C. and Edgerton, R. B. (eds.): *Changing Perspectives in Mental Illness*, New York.

Scheff, T. J. (1966), *Being Mentally Ill: A Sociological Theory*, Chicago.

Scheff, T. J. (ed.) (1967), *Mental Illness and Social Processes*, New York.

Schoenfeld, C. G. (1983), An Analysis of the Views of Thomas Szasz, in Vatz, R. E. and Weinberg, L. S. (eds.): *Thomas Szasz: Primary Values and Major Contentions*, New York.

Scull, A. T. (1979), *Museums of Madness: The Social Organization of Insanity in Nineteenth-Century England*, London.

Sedgwick, P. (1981), Illness - Mental and Otherwise, in Caplan, A.L., Engelhardt, H. T., Jr. and McCartney, J. J. (eds.): *Concepts of Health and Disease*, Reading, Massachusetts.

de Sousa, R. B. (1977), The Politics of Mental Illness, in *Inquiry*, 15, 1-2.

Svensson, T. (1994), *Residual Deviance, Insanity Ascription and Social Order*, Studies on Health and Society no. 22, Department of Health and Society, Linköping University.

Szasz, T. (1967), The Myth of Mental Illness, in Scheff, T. J. (ed.): *Mental Illness and Social Processes*, New York.

Szasz, T. (1974), *The Myth of Mental Illness*, New York, (revised edition).

Szasz, T. (1976), Schizophrenia: The Sacred Symbol of Psychiatry, in *British Journal of Psychiatry*, 129, pp. 308-316.

Szasz, T. (1981), The Concept of Mental Illness: Explanation or Justification, in Caplan, A. L., Engelhardt, H. T., Jr. and McCartney, J. J. (eds.): *Concepts of Health and Disease*, Reading, Massachusetts.

Turbayne, T. M. (1962), *The Myth of Metaphor*, New Haven.

Whitbeck, C. (1981), A Theory of Health, in Caplan, A. L., Engelhardt, H. T., Jr. and McCartney, J. J. (eds.): *Concepts of Health and Disease*, Reading, Massachusettts.

Index of names